Looking Good
from the Inside Out

fashion

Tammy Bennett

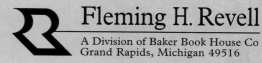

Fleming H. Revell
A Division of Baker Book House Co
Grand Rapids, Michigan 49516

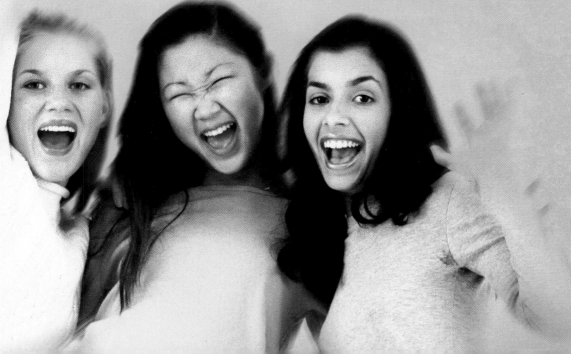

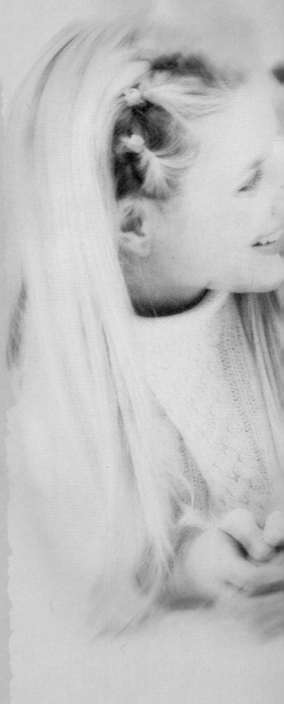

Published by Fleming H. Revell
a division of Baker Book House Company
P.O. Box 6287, Grand Rapids, MI 49516-6287
www.bakerbooks.com

Printed in the United States of America

Library of Congress Cataloging-in-Publication Data

Bennett, Tammy.
    Looking good from the inside out—fashion / Tammy Bennett.
        p.   cm.
    ISBN 0-8007-5887-0 (pbk.)
    1. Teenage girls—Religious life. 2. Clothing and dress—
Religious aspects—Christianity. I. Title.
    BV4551.3.B46 2003
    646'.34—dc21   2003007210

Cover design: Cheryl Van Andel

Interior design: Robin Black, UDG DesignWorks, Sisters, Oregon, www.udgdesignworks.com

Whisper Loud photo: ©Tony Baker Photography/Merge Left Reps, Inc.

Fashion photos pp. 42–42, 73, 76, 87, 114–116 by Stephen Gardner, His Image Pixelworks

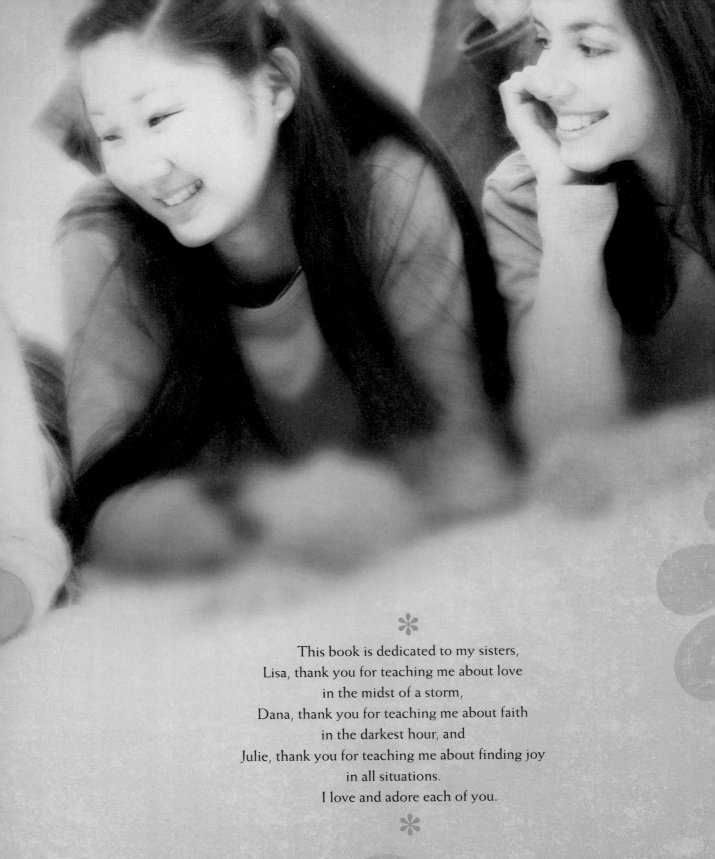

This book is dedicated to my sisters,
Lisa, thank you for teaching me about love
in the midst of a storm,
Dana, thank you for teaching me about faith
in the darkest hour, and
Julie, thank you for teaching me about finding joy
in all situations.
I love and adore each of you.

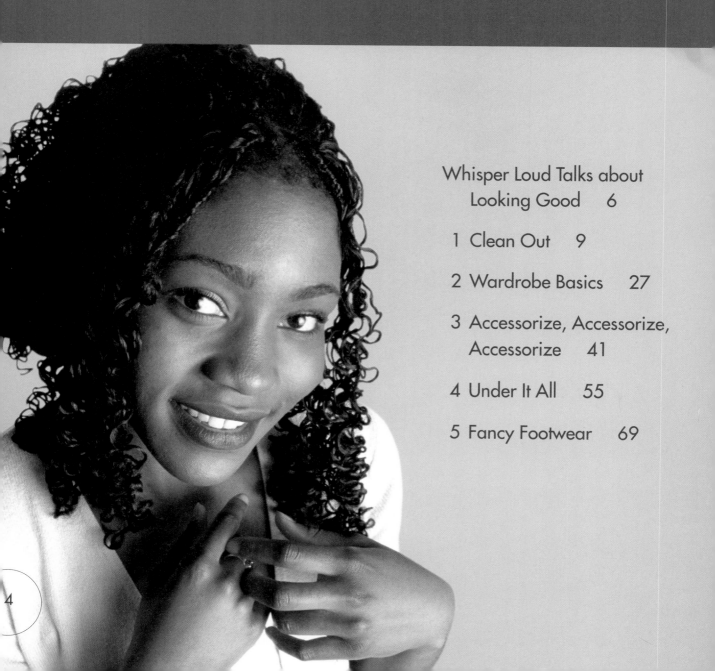

Contents

4

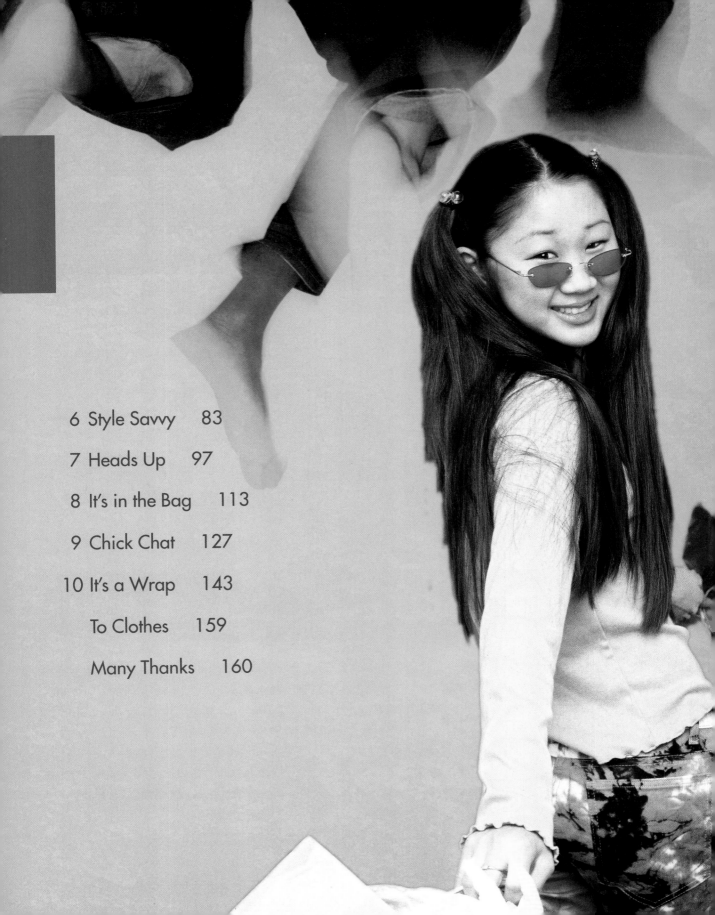

I had the pleasure of meeting the *Whisper Loud* gals, Tessa Gaskill, Keri Blumer, and Alana Carris, not long ago in New Orleans. With vibrant energy radiating from the inside out, these best friends, who have been singing together since childhood, represent what their hit song lyrically translates—*"A Different Kind of Beautiful."*

Please join me in getting to know these three Super (role) Models better.

TAMMY: Wow! This is so cool. Thanks for the interview. First off, as singing artists, what is the one thing you hope to convey to your listeners?

TESSA: We want our actions to speak louder than our words, which is actually where our name *Whisper Loud* comes from.

TAMMY: Since this book is about fashion, and the music industry promotes fashion, what can you tell us about how the two relate to you and each other?

Tessa: Music and fashion do go together. Every artist out there promotes some sort of look, whether they mean to or not. That's why it's important to us to dress in a way that doesn't compromise our values or faith.

Alana: We do take our responsibility as role models very seriously, and therefore we want to show girls how they can dress cool and be covered at the same time. They need to understand that you don't have to compromise modesty to be stylish.

Tammy: That is so true, but with the styles the way they are today, how do you choose trendy clothes that keep you covered up?

Keri: I allow my wardrobe to express who I am in a very cool and modest way. For example, I wear a long, thin undershirt under midriff tops, which I think looks more fashionable than wearing just one short shirt.

Tessa: I ask myself, "How will this affect my testimony in Christ?" If I have any doubts about the way it fits, I don't wear it and find something else.

Tammy: Can you give any specifics on how you dress with God in mind?

Alana: It all comes down to what we wear on the inside. Clothe yourself in the armor of God (truth, righteousness, peace, faith, salvation, Bible, and prayer), and you'll be able to combat the lies of the devil, live a better life, and feel better about yourself.

Whisper Loud Talks

Tammy: What a great lead-in to what this book is all about—looking good from the inside out, fashion for the body and soul. As we wrap up this interview, are there any last words of advice you'd like to share?

Alana: I love fashion, because it's one major way that a girl can reflect the kind of person she is and what she stands for, and hopefully after girls read this book, they'll take a stand for Christ.

Keri: I don't know if you're like me or not, but I like to be the one who stands out and starts new trends instead of just following the crowd. My advice is to be yourself—God made you in his image and he is perfect.

Tessa: How you dress yourself on the inside sticks out to people more than what you wear on the outside. Let people see the real you by letting Jesus shine through, and share a different kind of beautiful.

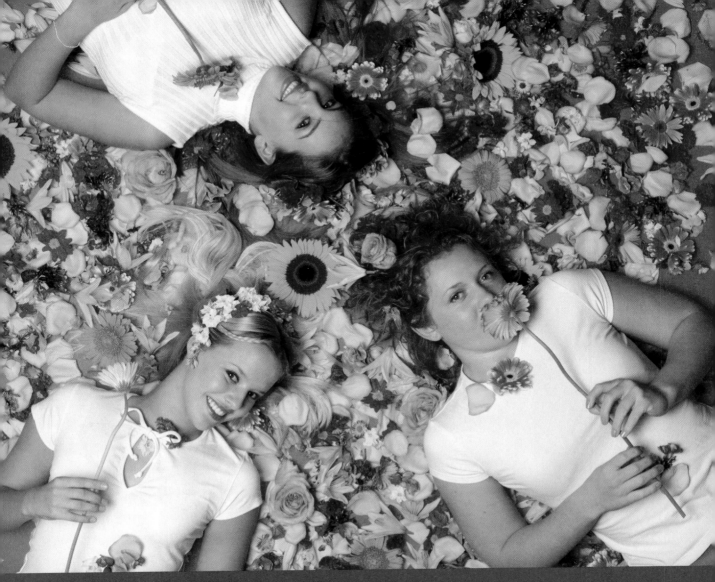

about Looking Good

Who we are goes into what we wear and who we want to be. In this book we'll review fashion trends and how they interpret who you are on the inside. We'll learn how to successfully dress from the inside out by looking underneath the clothes to the nitty-gritty heart of the matter. Girlfriends, we're going to learn how to dress with the soul in mind!

Tammy Bennett

For more information on *Whisper Loud* visit their web site: www.Whisperloud.com

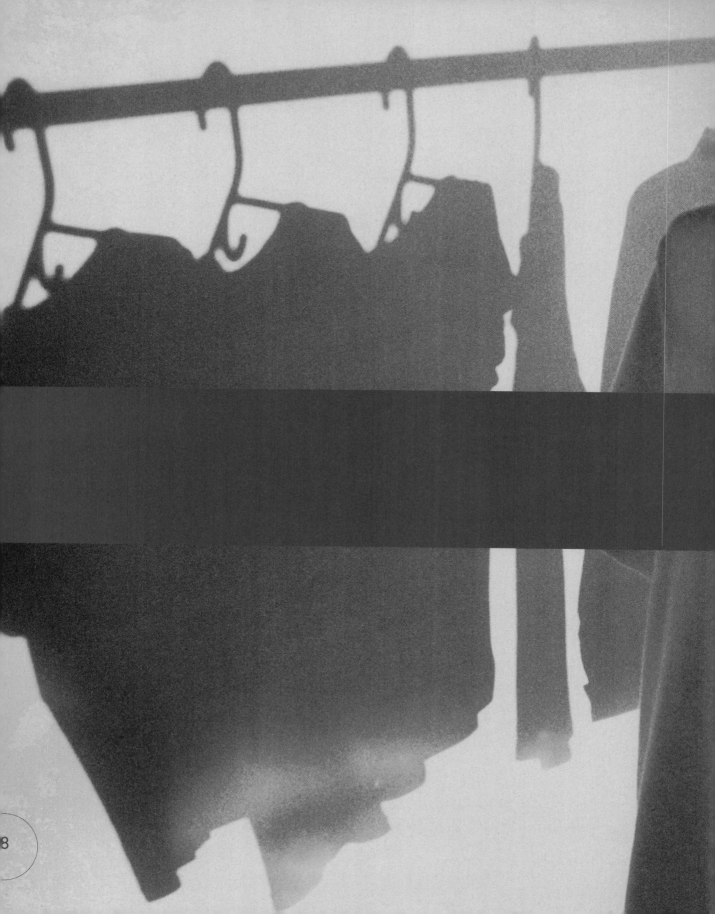

Clean Out

Part One—
Clean Out Your Closet

UGH! The mere thought of cleaning out the closet overwhelms me! Yet accomplishing anything takes work—including looking good. I fantasize about waking up, putting makeup on, setting my hair in place, and laying out my clothes so I can face the day in style. Then I wake up and reality sets in. I have puffy eyes and ratty

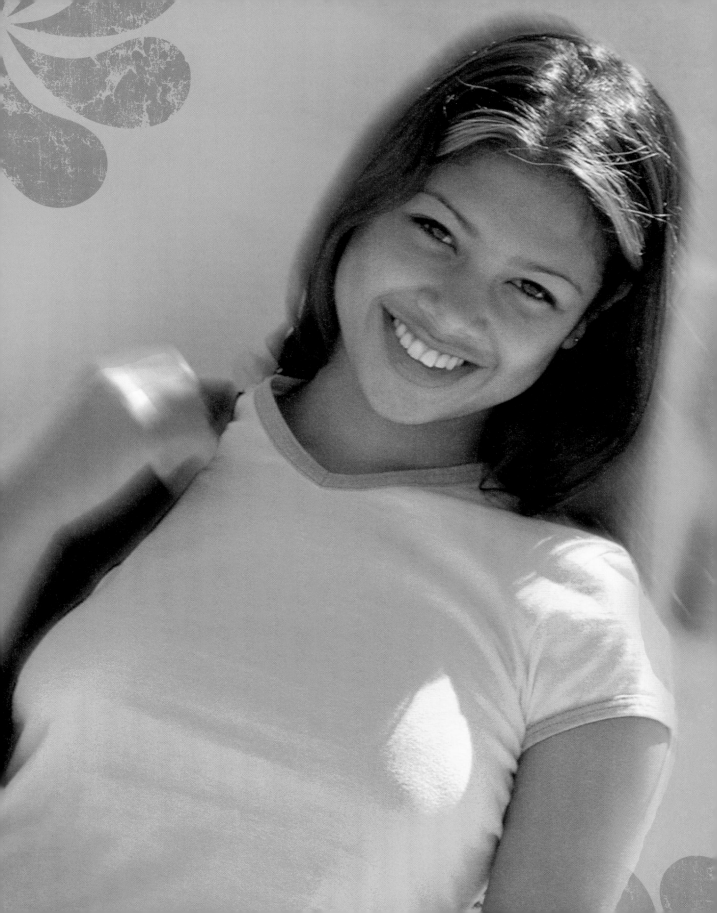

hair, and I can't find a thing to wear that makes me feel confident about the way I'm put together. ✳ Fortunately, those mornings have gotten fewer and farther between as I've learned to get a grip on fashion. I've discovered that creating a new style begins with cleaning out the closet. It's a big task, but don't despair. With a little know-how and the help of a friend you'll be dressing for success in no time.

The best place to start working on your wardrobe is in your own closet. Buried in the avalanche of clothes you will probably find some treasures. But to find those gems, you need to stand back, pull everything out of the closet, and carefully examine what's inside. This idea might sound unbearable, but think of it this way—you'll have a whole new wardrobe when you're through.

To make it less taxing and more entertaining, invite a friend over, crank up some music, and have fun. Once your closet inventory has been taken, go to your friend's house and do the same thing. And when you're finished, reward yourselves with a day of shopping to fill in your wardrobe gaps.

But let's not get too hasty, first things first. Get those trash bags in hand and let's get started.

Beware of the Door

Should "Open at Your Own Risk" be posted on the front of your closet door? Can you even begin to imagine what you'll find inside? "I haven't worn that since fourth

Out with the old. On with new style!

grade, and I never wore this ugly shirt my mother bought; the tags are still on it. Look at this, would you? I lost the other half of this two-piece swimsuit years ago, and my foot has grown at least two sizes since I last wore those shoes."

Similar thoughts will probably pop into your head as you start rummaging through your clothes collection. You're certain to get a good laugh, a sentimental memory, and an embarrassing thought about how ridiculous you must have looked as you rediscover garments from the past.

❋ Simple Solutions

As you clean your closet, you'll need to know what to keep and what to toss. Sounds easy, doesn't it? But it's more complicated than it sounds—if it were simple you wouldn't be in this fashion fix in the first place. Ready? Take a deep breath and let's get started.

Step #1—Sort by Season

Start with the current season. For example, let's say it's summer. Pull out all of your summer clothes and use the following steps to figure out what stays and what goes.

Step #2—Does It Fit?

This is a no-brainer. Try it on and look in the mirror. Does it pucker where it's not supposed to? Is it too short? Are you bulging at the seams? Can you sit down? Bend over? Breathe? Ask your friend for an *honest* opinion.

Step #3—Is It My Color?

Do you wear the color or does the color wear you? When you wear the right colors you look fresh and healthy; the colors flatter your natural skin tone. To determine colors that are good for you, think about the compliments others pay you, such as, "That color looks great on you!" or "You look particularly good today." When you're wearing the wrong color, you may hear comments like, "Are you feeling okay?" and "You look really tired." Remember this: Just because a color looks good on your best friend doesn't mean it will look good on you. My girlfriend Rose looks gorgeous in olive green, but when I put it on I look like death—nauseatingly green from head to toe!

Each of us has a particular set of colors that look best on us. Determining this "color season" can be kind of tricky but with a little know-how you'll easily discover your best colors. Color seasons are divided into two categories, warm or cool. Members of the "warm" family have a natural skin color with gold undertones, and members of the "cool" have a natural skin color with blue undertones. To determine whether you're "warm" or "cool" follow this simple test. Remove all makeup from your face and put your hair up in a white towel,

> Once you've discovered your **colors**, make shopping for them simple by carrying paint samples (located in the paint department of your local hardware store) of them in your purse or wallet.

carefully removing all traces of hair from around your face. Then use either shiny gold fabric or a large piece of gold jewelry (such as a large earring), hold it close to your face, and observe what you see in the mirror. Make the same observations using shiny silver fabric or a larger piece of silver jewelry.

1. Which one makes your face appear the most red and blotchy? Gold or silver?
2. Which one makes your skin appear creamier and less blotchy? Gold or silver?

If you answered *gold* in question number one and *silver* for the second question, then you are a member of the "cool" family. If you answered *silver* for the first question and *gold* for the second, you're a member of the "warm" family.

Which are you? (circle one)   WARM   or   COOL

If you're a member of the "warm" family then your colors will be either "autumn" or "spring." Both of these color seasons contain gold undertones but they have different color intensity. Autumn colors are made up of rich, dark shades of brown, rust, olive, orange, orange red, and creamy white. Spring has a lighter color value with bright hues of browns, rust, olive, orange, orange red, and tan. To determine your season, hold an assortment of colors from the autumn (rich and dark) and spring (light and bright) families up to your makeup-free face and toweled head and select the one that works best with your skin tone. If you can't decide on your own, ask your mom or a friend for their opinion.

Autumn   Spring

Members of the "cool" family fall into the "winter" or "summer" seasons. Winter colors are made up of rich, dark shades of gray, purple, navy blue, blue red, and bright white. If you're a winter person, one of your best colors is classic black. Summer colors have subtle tints of the winter color palette; light gray, a hint of purple, soft blue gray, pink, berry red, and white. To determine your season, hold an assortment of colors from the winter (rich and dark) and summer (soft and subtle) families up to your makeup-free face and toweled head and select the one that works best with your skin tone. Remember to ask for help if you can't decide on your own.

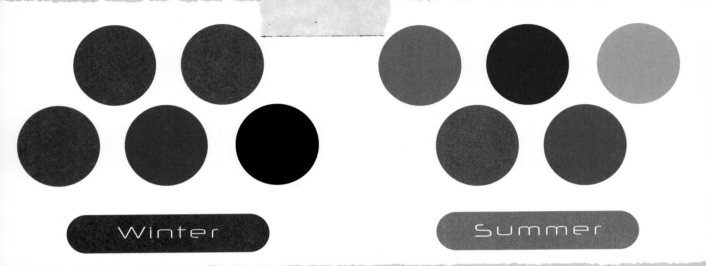

Winter   Summer

If you are still baffled by this color thing, try reading books by Color Me Beautiful (check on Color Me Beautiful's web site) or hire a professional color consultant to determine your color palette.

Step #4—Is It Flattering to My Figure?

To get a clear-cut look at your wardrobe, you'll have to take your body shape into consideration. Are your clothes tailored to fit you in all the right places? Do they enhance the positive and erase the negative? Do they flatter your figure? Did you buy it with your body shape in mind or was it purchased on a whim because it looked great on the store mannequin?

I've yet to see anyone with the shape of a mannequin, but we're often coaxed into spending big bucks on clothes that look remarkable on their fictitious bodies. Did you know that it is absolutely impossible for anyone to be the size and shape of a mannequin and still have properly functioning organs? I wish stores would have models that look like real people rather than using dummies that are ill-proportioned. Shopping would be much easier if we could see clothes modeled on a realistic mannequin!

Fortunately, you can look like a living, breathing store mannequin when you wear clothes designed to work with your body type. Once you learn the shape of your body, you can flatter your figure by wearing the right clothing. Read through the examples below to determine which body shape sounds the most like your own and then apply the dressing directions for your specific body type. It may sound confusing at first, but with some practice your wardrobe will be well-balanced in no time.

Pear Shape—

Object: Create visual balance by enhancing the top and downplaying the bottom.

If you've been blessed with a pear-shaped body, your top is proportionally smaller than your bottom. In order to create visual balance you need to accentuate your top half and downplay your bottom. Two quick fixes are shoulder pads (but not too big!) and the infamous padded bra. You can also try wearing a scarf, jacket, or cardigan sweater. Just make sure the jacket or sweater hangs down to or below your widest area. When choosing skirts, pants, or jeans, the trick is to find some that are not too tight around the hips or too big around the waist. If faced with this challenge, pick one that fits around the hips rather than the waist and then camouflage the larger waistband with a sweater or blouse. Try this on for size. Wear a top with volume to it, such as a ruffled blouse or bulky sweater, with a slim fitting (not tight) skirt, pants, or jeans.

Rectangular Shape—

Object: Create visual balance by contouring the waistline.

The rectangle body shape has shoulders and hips that are about the same width and a waistline that doesn't vary more than a few inches. To create dimension, you should create the illusion of a tapered waistline. Try wearing a shirt tucked into a skirt, pants, or jeans with a belted, low-rise waistband. Complete the look with a jacket or cardigan that hangs below the waist.

Apple Shape—

Object: Create visual balance by drawing attention away from the waistline.

The apple body shape is round and short-waisted without a well-defined figure. Loose fitting, solid-colored garments look best on this body shape. Use shoulder pads to draw the eye away from your waistline. When choosing skirts, pants, or jeans, stay away from pleats that can make you look larger. Try wearing a boxy blouse or jacket that hangs in a straight line from your shoulders to just below your bottom.

Hourglass Shape—

Object: Accentuate your natural curves and waistline.

The hourglass figure is the most balanced of all body types. It has wide shoulders, a defined bustline, narrow waist (the waistline is approximately ten inches smaller than the bust and hips), and rounded hips. Your goal when dressing is to accentuate your waist. Wear clothing with rounded shoulders and necklines designed in solid colors or rounded prints to accentuate your natural curves. Avoid loose, baggy clothing and striped or plaid fabrics—they will make you look chubby. If you are short, you do not want to wear prints that are large and overpowering to your height. A terrific look for the hourglass shape is a shirt or blouse with a crossover neckline tucked into a skirt, pants, or jeans.

Wedge Shape—

Object: Create balance by visually softening the angular body shape.

The wedge figure or upside-down triangle has an athletic, boyish look with broad shoulders that taper down into a narrow waist and straight legs. Your best look is made up of tailored, solid colors or crisp, angular prints that flatter your figure. But you should avoid wearing shoulder pads. An awesome outfit for you is a shirt tucked into a low-rise, soft-pleated bottom with a wide belt.

Step #5—When Was the Last Time You Wore It?

Have you worn the item once in the last year? If you haven't, chances are you never will. One exception to this rule applies to formal attire. If you have a fancy outfit that you haven't worn in awhile but know you'll wear again, then keep it.

I have the most difficulty with this rule. I'll get on a cleaning binge and start dumping anything in my wardrobe that I haven't worn in awhile, but then as the binge subsides I grow weak and start reclaiming the castoffs, hoping to wear them someday. Of course "someday" never comes, and those clothes hang untouched awaiting my next cleaning binge. Trust me. If you haven't worn something in one full year, you won't wear it again unless you plan to rejuvenate it. Do yourself a favor and get rid of it only once.

Step #6—Can It Be Renewed?

Does the item in question have any redeemable value? Would you wear it again with updated accessories such as a new belt, buttons, or jewelry? What about mixing and matching it with other pieces in your closet?

This is where the expertise of a friend becomes extremely useful. Ask your fashion buddy to shop your closet for some fresh wardrobe ideas. We often overlook brand-new outfits waiting at our fingertips. It takes someone with a fresh approach to discover what you've become oblivious to. You might buy a shirt and shorts as an outfit, never dreaming of mixing and matching them with other pieces. When a friend suggests that you wear a different belt with that combination, you have a new outfit!

Another way you might refurbish clothing is by dyeing it. If you've tried something on that's really not your color, ask yourself this question: "Would it be something I would wear if it was the right color?" If the answer is yes then buy some Rit fabric dye (follow the directions on the box) and change the color to match your skin tone. Recently I found a faded T-shirt in my drawer. It needed something if I was ever going to wear it again, so I decided to spruce it up a little. For just a few dollars I redyed it and added a few sequins. Now it looks better than new! There are many ways you can recycle boring basics into fabulous fashions. Turn a tired T-shirt into a trendy top. Jazz up junky jeans. Spruce up sorry socks. Overhaul overalls. Be creative. Lace, ribbon, fringe, buttons, belts, rhinestones, pins, flowers, jewelry, fabric paint, patches, appliqués—the possibilities are endless!

> Every body shape is positively accentuated with good **posture**. Practice good posture by standing and sitting up straight.

Okay, now that you have made it this far, the next assignment is easy. Gather four trash bags, boxes, or other containers labeled Trash, Toss, Trade, and Touch-Up.

Trash: Trash it in the garbage can. I don't know how many times I have saved holey T-shirts or ripped jeans thinking that I might wear them to paint in someday. They never got worn and are still hoarding much-needed closet space. And of course there are those pieces with sentimental value. "I love that blue blouse. I was asked out on my first date while wearing it." That may sound like reason enough to cherish it, but if you've outgrown it, it's fraying at the seams, and you wouldn't be caught dead in it, why are you keeping it? Get over the sentiments, have an official burial, and throw it away!

Toss: Toss it into the donation pile. These are items that still have life left in them, but you'll never wear them again and neither would your friends. Write down each item you toss as well as a reasonable dollar value so you or your parents can receive the tax benefit for charitable donations. There are many charities that would welcome your left-over clothing. Ask a local church, or look in your phone book for charitable organizations.

Trade: Trade it with your friends. Maybe you have outgrown it, or it's one of those purchases that looked good on the hanger but didn't look good once you got it home. Or maybe your mom bought it for you and it's just not your taste. Whatever the case, it might be just what your friend was looking for. This is the fun part. Host a hand-me-down party. After you and your friends have cleaned out your closets, get together with your trade piles and trade with one another. Avoid hurt feelings by drawing names for the popular items that are wanted by more than one person. When you're finished, donate the leftovers to a charity.

Touch-Up: If you have clothes that you plan to spruce up, put them in the touch-up bag and schedule a time to do the touch-up work. What can you do to fix up what's in this box? Keep in mind that if you need help, you can always find assistance at fabric and craft stores.

> If you have not worn it in one year, chances are you never will, so **file it** in the appropriate container.

Time Out
with Tammy

I'm crazy about hand-me-downs! Now don't get me wrong. I have a weakness for new clothes too, but secondhand clothing will always bring fond memories to mind; those of Diane (one of my lifelong buds), in-house fashion shows, and Donny Osmond.

I loved new clothes when I was growing up, but since I was the oldest of five they were not always affordable. Often the oldest gets new stuff that's handed down to younger siblings, but even though I was the oldest, I still received hand-me-downs from my friend. Every Saturday Diane and her parents came over to visit for the evening. Just before their scheduled arrival I would perch myself in front of the window, hoping to spot brown paper bags. If Diane arrived with grocery bags in tote, I was getting new clothes. I would race out, greet them at the curb, grab the bags, and race into the house. Once inside, Diane would stack *Donny Osmond's Greatest Hits* onto the record player while I changed into one of my new outfits. I'd use my bed as a runway and model my new apparel. I'd pivot and turn, smile and wave, and feel like Miss America in my new-to-me clothing.

Take it from me. There is nothing wrong with secondhand clothing. It doesn't matter if it's given to you or if you purchase it, you'll still feel first-class when you wear it.

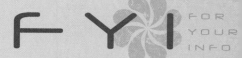

Did you know that what may be worthless to you might be worth big bucks to someone else? There is money to be made with used clothing and accessories. Have you ever checked out Ebay? I love shopping Ebay for used clothing. I can find the same things online that I find in catalogues and malls, at a fraction of the price.

My sister-in-law often buys bargain clearance clothes in stores and sells them on Ebay at a profit. Either way you look at it, you just can't go wrong. If you're selling, you're able to determine your minimum-selling price ahead of time; and if you're buying, you can bid your maximum and hope for the best.

Important Note: Ask your parents' or guardian's permission to use Ebay or any other online auction before you begin.

❋ What This Means 2U

Out with the old, in with new style! You are on your way to a new attitude about getting dressed. For most of us, it's not a matter of *if* we have clothes to wear—most of our closets and drawers are jam-packed—it's a matter of whether our clothes make us feel good about the way we look. Once you clean out what doesn't fit and flatter and find fashionable outfits you didn't even know you had, you'll look and feel more confident as an individual.

Don't take this the wrong way. Dressing for success won't change who you are on the inside. If you lie, cheat, steal, and do drugs, a new look won't ease your conscience. It'll just hide the rags of your character that lie beneath the surface. Not sure what I'm talking about? Then please read on and join me in part 2 of this chapter.

Test It Out

Have you started cleaning out your closets and drawers yet? Are you amazed at how much you can get rid of? Are you suffering from separation anxiety? Well, you'll be happy to know that the hard part is over. Now it's time to get the proper containers to the proper places. Trash it, Toss it, Trade it, or Touch-Up.

When you're finished, you'll feel better. Cleaning out always makes me feel like I've accomplished something significant. Whether it's a matter of cleaning out my socks drawer or digging a little deeper into the drawer of my heart, a fresh start always does wonders for who I am outside and inside.

Cluttered closets leave you clueless, but cleaned-out closets lead to clothes you can feel **confident** in.

What Color Is Your Shape?

Which color family do you belong in?

Warm   Cool

Which color season looks best on you?

Autumn   Spring   Winter   Summer

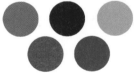

What is your body shape?

Pear   Rectangle   Apple   Hourglass   Wedge

Take note of your personal color season and body shape because as you read through the book I'm going to teach you how to have fun, take control, and rebuild your wardrobe with your needs in mind.

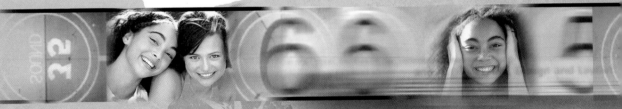

Part Two—Clean Out the Closet of Your Heart

Creating a new wardrobe and a new you begins with cleaning out the junk that's been buried in your closet for years. There are usually a lot of "has been" or "never were" articles of clothing that you should have gotten rid of long ago. But as long as they were buried deep within the closet or stashed under your bed, you didn't have to deal with them. Out of sight, out of mind. ✳ How many of us have lives that resemble the same mess? But instead of clothes that need to be cleaned out, we have sins that need to be cleared out of our hearts. We need a fresh new start with Jesus, the only answer to dealing with sin. When you invite Jesus into your life, he cleans out the closet of your soul and makes room for the Holy Spirit to abide in you. He gives you a new look from the inside out.

Psalm 139:15–16 (MESSAGE)—You know exactly how I was made, bit by bit, how I was sculpted from nothing into something. Like an open book, you watched me grow from conception to birth; all the stages of my life were spread out before you, the days of my life all prepared before I'd even lived one day.

How cool is that? God knew us before we were ever born. Don't you think it's time that you got acquainted with him? If you have not met him yet, please allow me the honor of introducing Jesus Christ to you.

Revelation 3:20 (NKJV)—Behold, I stand at the door and knock. If anyone hears My voice and opens the door, I will come in to [her] and dine with [her], and [she] with Me.

Wow! Are you ready for this kind of life-changing relationship? All you have to do is open the door to your soul by asking Jesus to come into your life, and he will become your faithful companion. But beware! If you ignore the knocking you are risking it all.

❊ Soulful Solutions

First things first. No rules, regulations, or religion can equal a relationship with Jesus Christ. He'll love and accept you just the way you are, but you need to open the door of your heart and ask him in. It may sound complicated at first, but in reality it's very simple. If you are ready for this kind of companionship, then read on.

I can only imagine what you may be thinking right now. "Who me? God would never forgive me for what I've done." "If God really loved me he wouldn't let such bad things happen to me." "I could never be good enough to be a Christian." "Christians don't have any fun." Do any of these statements sound at all like the thoughts running through your mind about now?

Well, let me put your thoughts at ease. God will forgive you for whatever you have done. He will give you the strength to endure anything you're up against. He doesn't expect perfection (that's exactly why he provided us with perfection through a relationship in his Son, Jesus!). And whoever told you Christians don't have fun was just plain WRONG!

Scripture It

Jesus is waiting for you to accept his invitation to come into your life and sweep you off your feet. Just believe his Word with no exceptions and choose to open the door to the closet of your soul. He can't wait to make your dreams come true.

Trash

Romans 3:23 (NKJV)—For all have sinned and fall short of the glory of God.

Our sin is like trash in the eyes of God. The sight of it repulses him, the smell of it disgusts him, and the fact that we clutter our hearts and lives with it separates us from having a relationship with him.

> Jesus will strip you of your sin and **outfit you** with new life.

Everyone has done something wrong at one time or another. Being a sinner doesn't mean you robbed a bank or killed somebody. It may just mean you lied to your mom, cheated on a test, or hit your annoying brother. We've all stunk up and cluttered our lives with trashy sin; so what do we do with the garbage? It has to be taken out, and God provided his Son, Jesus Christ, to do just that. When we ask Jesus to take the trash out, he clears the sin and makes us clean inside so we can spend eternity in heaven with God.

Toss

Ephesians 2:8–9 (NKJV)—For by grace you have been saved through faith, and that not of yourselves; it is the gift of God, not of works, lest anyone should boast .

Toss out the idea that you can earn your way to heaven. Remember when I said there is nothing God could not forgive you for? Well, the opposite is also true; there is nothing you can do that is good enough either. Your only claim to eternal life with God is to accept his gift (Jesus) by inviting him into your life.

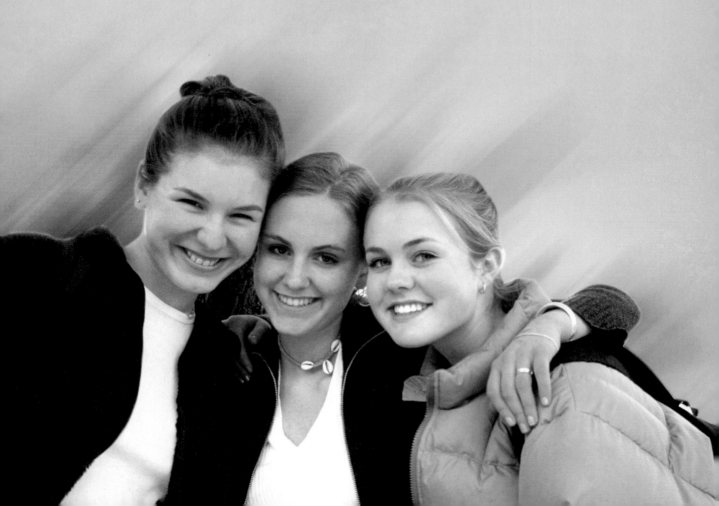

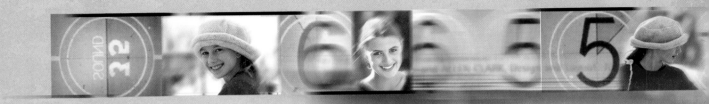

Trade

John 3:16 (NKJV)—For God so loved the world that He gave His only begotten Son, that whoever believes in Him should not perish but have everlasting life.

God traded the life of his Son for your salvation. It's that simple. God loves you so much that he sent his Son to die on the cross for your sins. It only requires acceptance on your part to have a relationship with Jesus Christ and have the sin cleaned out of your heart.

Touch-Up

Will you ask Jesus into your life so he can touch up your soul? It's all up to you now. Either invite him into your life or ignore his knocking. When you ask Christ, he'll clean out the sinful garbage from your soul and abide with you throughout all eternity. Are you ready for a relationship with Jesus? He's ready for a relationship with you.

Below is a prayer that will help you. Reciting this prayer off the top of your head a million times won't do you any good unless you make it personal between you and God. So be real. Invite Jesus into your life.

> Dear Lord,
>
> I know that I am a sinner and that I can't do anything about it on my own. Through faith I believe that you sent your Son, Jesus, to die for my sins, that he was buried and rose again, and that I can have eternal life through a relationship with him. I accept your gift of salvation and trust in you to be Lord of my life.
>
> In Jesus' Name, Amen.

No rules, regulations, or religion can = **a relationship** with Jesus.

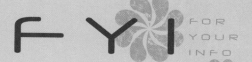

FOR
YOUR
INFO

Now that Jesus has come into your life and cleaned out the sin, the Holy Spirit has moved in to guide you every day of your life. You're no longer going it alone. Through thick and thin, good and bad; the Holy Spirit will get you through it all if you will rely on him.

Ephesians 1:13–14 (MESSAGE)—*It's in Christ that you, once you heard the truth and believed it (this Message of your salvation), found yourselves home free—signed, sealed, and delivered by the Holy Spirit. This signet from God is the first installment on what's coming, a reminder that we'll get everything God has planned for us, a praising and glorious life.*

Time Out
with Tammy

You're not the only one that wonders about spiritual things. Many girls have the very same questions as you when they are introduced to Jesus.

Tiffany was one who asked all those questions and more. I met her several years ago when I was a camp counselor for junior high girls. I arrived at the camp early in the morning, unpacked, and set up my cabin just before the girls began trickling in. One by one they arrived, claimed their bunk, hauled in their luggage, and hugged their parents good-bye. At the appointed time I gave roll call, checking off each girl on my list. But one girl was absent. I made note of it and rallied the rest of the girls together for the first big camp event, dinner.

Once we stepped out of the cabin, I spied Tiffany sitting on the porch step, slouched over and clinging to her green camouflage duffle bag. I didn't know what to make of her at first but the collective gasp of the other girls said it all.

She was dressed in black from head to toe, with dyed black hair, black nail polish, and black lip and eyeliner. She instantly shot me the "I don't want to be here look" and turned away. I passed her without saying a word and directed the rest of the cabin to the dining hall.

Once I bid them farewell I turned to Tiffany to welcome her to camp. She looked up at me with angry tears filling her eyes and said she wanted to go home. I told her she should give the place a chance before she made any hasty decisions and invited her into the cabin to get settled. Once inside she plopped her body and bag onto the bed. I invited her to walk with me to dinner and headed for the door. The moment the screen door shut behind me she screamed out, "I hate this place, I hate you, I hate my parents, and I hate myself!"

Here was a girl full of anger, hurt, and rejection. She didn't know what it was to feel unconditional love

24

Congratulations! Please allow me to be the first to welcome you into the family of God. I'd love to hear all about it! (You can drop me a note at: MakeOverMin@aol.com.)

❋ What This Means 2U

Wow! Once you've asked Jesus into your life, God impresses his signet ring upon your heart and marks you as an official daughter of the King of kings. You are a genuine *princess!* And God has given you the Holy Spirit to guide and direct your every step—a still, small voice that lies deep within you and prompts you to do the right thing.

> *Galatians 5:16—Live by the Spirit, and you will not gratify the desires of the sinful nature.*

◗ Test It Out

Cleaning out is the biggest step you will take for both your wardrobe and your soul. When you clean out your heart and your closet, you'll gain a fresh lease on life. When you clear away the junk you've collected in your drawers and the sin you've accumulated in your life, you make way for a new you, both body and soul.

Super Models **clean** from the inside out.

because her only acceptance came from the gang she belonged to. Tiffany found it hard to believe she could experience forgiveness because she participated in illegal gang activities. "Robbery, rape, rituals—I'm too bad to go to heaven," she said. I had to admit she had been wrapped up in some pretty heavy stuff, but I told her that a God who is merciful doesn't judge us according to our past sin but according to the forgiveness we receive through a relationship with Jesus Christ. Tiffany invited Jesus into her life that afternoon and hasn't been the same since.

The black wardrobe, hair, and makeup have disappeared, and she's found real love and acceptance through a relationship with Jesus. Leaving the gang wasn't easy—in fact it was life-threatening. But God helped her through the transition, and now she's helping other girls find real acceptance outside of gangs and within the parameters of a loving relationship with Jesus Christ.

Does this sound too much like a fairy tale to you? Once upon a time . . . she lived happily ever after. Well, this is not make-believe, this is reality. You are the heroine of the story, awaiting your prince (Jesus) to save you from the fire-breathing dragon (Satan). But he won't come into your life unless you ask him in and agree to become his bride.

The "once upon a time" begins the moment you accept Christ into your life and the "happily ever after" will be eternity in heaven with God. So what happens in between? Your life, with all the ups and downs that lie ahead. Being a Christian won't make life easy, but trusting Jesus will help you brave all of life's storms. Like Tiffany, you too can face life's biggest challenges with Jesus by your side.

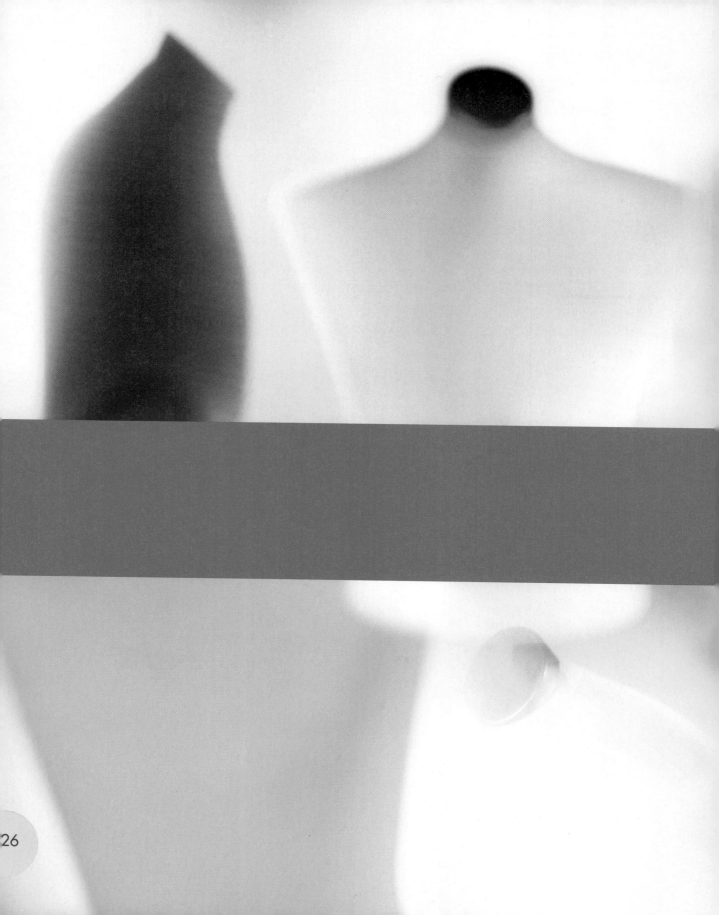

Wardrobe Basics

Part One–
Rebuild Your Wardrobe

Now that you've cleared out the old stuff, you're ready to rebuild, reorganize, and replenish your wardrobe. It's time to take a clothing inventory. We'll work our way through the basics in this chapter, and when we're finished, you'll know how to build your wardrobe starting with what you have on hand. ✳ You're on your way to becoming an official member of the "fashion police." As a clothing informant you'll be

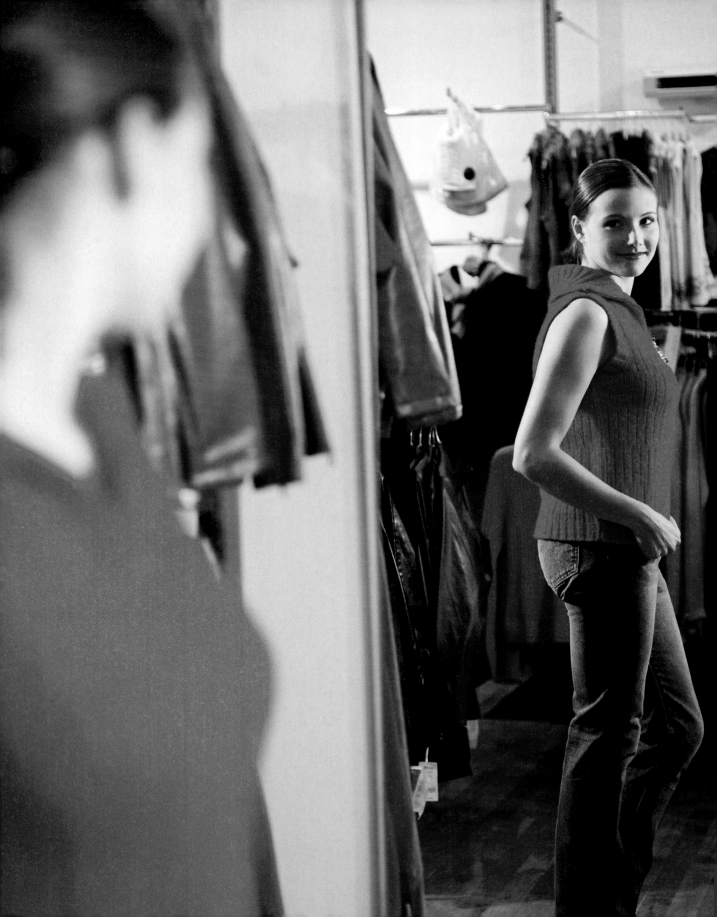

able to blow the whistle on mismanaged style according to the needs of your own life. You'll handcuff time restraints by coordinating color with style and crack down on poor spending by replenishing your wardrobe with wise purchases. ✳ Are you ready to get indoctrinated into this fashion academy? Let's get started!

I'm going to promote you to manager of your very own clothing boutique. As the boss you'll be in charge of taking inventory, maximizing space, arranging displays, and cleaning out clearance items. Additional responsibilities will include purchasing new merchandise and improving your marketing approach. With your new title you'll also receive a raise in your self-worth—you'll gain new confidence in the way you look and feel about yourself. So if you're ready to assume your duties, I'm ready to teach you the basics of clothing management.

A shop manager needs to name the store. I've named my shop "Tammy's Dressing Room," but there's still a lot to do before I'm officially open for business. The first item on a good manager's agenda should be rebuilding inventory. But where should we begin?

You might be thinking we should start in the lingerie department because we naturally dress from the inside out. But I prefer to begin with the outer garments and work my way in. After we pick our outside clothing, we can fill in our undergarments with the appropriate colors and styles. With this in mind, let's get to work.

Get a grip
on your
clothesline

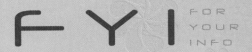

Are you still trying to find closet space and make room in your dresser drawers? Don't despair. There are many creative things you can do to increase your space. Below are some ideas that will help you economize space and may even inspire you to invent your own space-saving solutions.

Closet

Keep your shoes stored in their original boxes. Label them according to color and style and then stack them by color on the floor or on a shelf with the labeled end showing.

Closet shelving is a great way to store everything from T-shirts to toiletries. You can buy inexpensive shelving units at most home improvement stores or build your own.

Use stackable plastic bins to store things such as handbags, hats, and beachwear.

Clear plastic divided shoe bags are a great way to store not only shoes but also other smaller items such as hair accessories, jewelry, pantyhose, toiletries, and school supplies.

Keep your robe on a hook and your pj's under your pillow for easy access.

Use long nails or hooks to hang up hats, belts, handbags, and backpacks.

Place cedar blocks in your closet and dresser drawers to repel moths.

Drawers

Are your drawers too stuffed? Hang up your nighties.

Use small plastic baskets to separate socks and underwear.

Roll up shirts instead of folding them. This saves space and prevents wrinkles.

Extras

Use decorative hatboxes to store things in such as hats, belts, handbags, scarves, and hair accessories.

Store everything from sweaters to shoes in plastic, under-the-bed storage bins (found at most discount stores). Or increase your space with bed lifts (these can be found at most linen stores). They allow you to use regular-sized storage boxes and bins under your bed.

Use three-inch, three-ring binders to store smaller lightweight items, such as hose or hair barrettes. Take a Ziploc bag and punch holes in the bag on the opposite end of the closure and then insert it into the notebook. I store one pair of pantyhose in each bag and then use notebook dividers to separate the colors. This method makes it simple to pack hose; I just remove the Ziploc bag from the binder and put it in my suitcase.

Use a plastic, sectioned, fishing tackle box to store earrings.

Use a multi-tiered pants rack to hang belts or scarves .

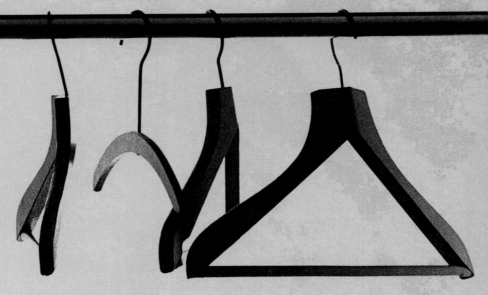

✳ Simple Solutions

There are three simple steps that will help you inventory, stock, rebuild, and maximize space in your wardrobe. Follow the directions below and you'll have your store open for business in no time.

Step #1—Reorganize

Organize your closet and dresser into sections by season, style, or both. The seasonal method divides your wardrobe into four seasons: summer, autumn, winter, and spring. The style method divides your wardrobe into categories: casual, athletic, beach, dress, formal, outerwear, and sleepwear. My dresser drawers are arranged by season. I have one drawer designated for winter pajamas, one for summer nighties, one for winter sweaters, one for summer shorts, and one for summer beachwear. On the other hand, my closet is divided into styles: formal wear, dressy wear, casual wear, and outerwear.

Step #2—Regroup and Rearrange

Separate articles in each section (season or style) so they are hanging in groups: pants with pants, blouses with blouses, and so on. Then arrange them by color. My closet is coordinated by category and color. For instance, my formal wear is divided into colors (blacks, grays, blues, purples, reds, and whites) and then categorized according to the item (dresses, skirts, shirts, and pants). My dressy and casual wear are divided the same way, but my outerwear (jackets and coats) are divided primarily by color.

Congratulations! You've conquered the first two steps. There's only one step left, but before we get to it, pull out your pen and notebook. It's time to take notes on what you have and what you need. We'll work our way through bare essentials, but first answer this question:

What type of lifestyle do you lead?

Home, work, school, activities, climate, and your own personal style—all of these factors will determine your answer. Just remember this one important point: Your wardrobe won't suit your personality or needs if you aren't honest with yourself. Don't describe the lifestyle you sometimes *pretend* to lead; be proud of who you really are.

Time Out
with Tammy

When I was younger, I was always busy trying to be someone else. I was never content with who I was, where I lived, and the activities I enjoyed. Instead, I wanted to be someone popular who lived in the big city and excelled at sports.

As you can imagine my wardrobe didn't meet my needs. I picked out popular name brands even when I didn't like the styles, thinking they would give me social status among my peers. I dressed with a big city in mind even though I grew up in the farmland. A lot of what I bought was impractical—it hung in my closet awaiting an opportunity to be worn. I also wasted money on athletic clothing because I thought it would make me sporty even though I hated participating in most sporting events. My wardrobe wasn't about who I was, it was about who I *wanted* to be. After awhile, I just wanted to return to reality and get into my own duds.

It's okay to be yourself. Allow your personality to shine through your clothing. If you like wearing jeans and T-shirts, then wear them. If you like dressing up, then don't feel intimidated, just do it. Always be yourself.

Step #3—Replenish

Now that you've considered your lifestyle, you can make a list of what you have and what you need. Start your list the same way you divided your wardrobe, by season and by style. Review your wardrobe in the current season because this is the one you will shop for first. What do you have on hand? What do you need? Do you need shorts or pants? Do you need tops? If so, what colors? What about your dressy wear, athletic wear, or beachwear? Is there anything missing? Add it to your list.

Now that your know what you'll be wearing on the outside, you can buy the appropriate color and style underwear. For instance if you have light-colored shirts, you will want to wear a natural-colored bra, never white, because it glows through most fabrics. If you wear a dark color then you'll want to wear a dark-colored bra to match. The same rule of thumb applies to your shorts, pants, or skirts when buying panties.

Consider which style underwear works best beneath your clothing. You don't want your bra or underwear to show; it's a matter of dressing with respect for yourself and others. The waistband of your underwear should not be seen hanging out above the waistband of your shorts, pants, or skirt and your bra should be fully contained beneath your top, straps and all. You should also think about undergarments for those special needs, such as tummy control underwear or athletic support bras. Whatever the need, be sure to write it down.

Reorganize, regroup, rearrange, and replenish a **renewed** you!

❱Test It Out

Do you have what it takes to be a member in good standing of the fashion police? Have you rebuilt your own shop efficiently so it saves you time and money? Keep in mind, a good wardrobe manager organizes her space so it works for her, she buys according to her own lifestyle, and she is always a prudent shopper. Use the form below to help you shop and fill in where your wardrobe is lacking.

DEFINE YOUR LIFESTYLE.

What do you prefer to wear and what are you most comfortable in at home?

What do you prefer to wear and what are you most comfortable in at school?

What extracurricular activities are you involved in and how do they affect your dress?

What do you consider to be your lifestyle?

CLOTHING INVENTORY

Write down what you need by Season:

    Summer:

    Autumn:

    Winter:

    Spring:

OR

Write down what you need by Style:

    Athletic:

    Beach:

    Casual:

    Dressy:

    Formal:

    Outer:

    Sleep:

    Lingerie:

Write down your body shape and color season.

    Body shape:

    Color season:

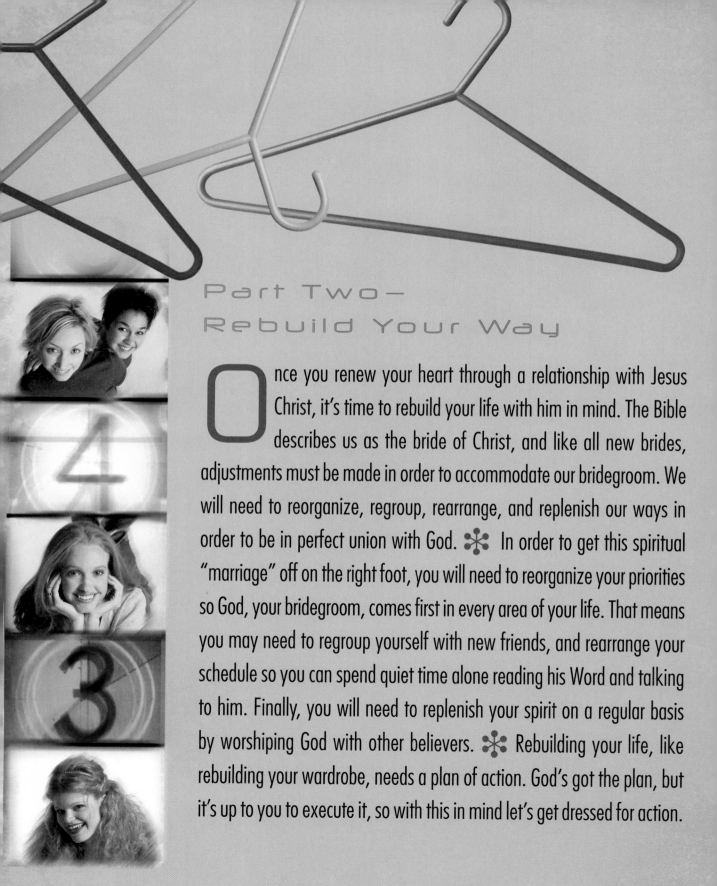

Part Two—
Rebuild Your Way

Once you renew your heart through a relationship with Jesus Christ, it's time to rebuild your life with him in mind. The Bible describes us as the bride of Christ, and like all new brides, adjustments must be made in order to accommodate our bridegroom. We will need to reorganize, regroup, rearrange, and replenish our ways in order to be in perfect union with God. ✳ In order to get this spiritual "marriage" off on the right foot, you will need to reorganize your priorities so God, your bridegroom, comes first in every area of your life. That means you may need to regroup yourself with new friends, and rearrange your schedule so you can spend quiet time alone reading his Word and talking to him. Finally, you will need to replenish your spirit on a regular basis by worshiping God with other believers. ✳ Rebuilding your life, like rebuilding your wardrobe, needs a plan of action. God's got the plan, but it's up to you to execute it, so with this in mind let's get dressed for action.

Part of the wedding tradition involves picking out a bridal gown. When a bride is dressing for her groom, she wants everything to be just right. Careful consideration goes into every single item she puts on, and she wants everything to be perfect for her main man, husband, provider, protector, and best friend.

God uses the marriage analogy to teach us about the special bond we have with him.

Ephesians 5:22,25–28 (MESSAGE)—Wives, understand and support your husbands in ways that show your support for Christ. . . . Husbands, go all out in your love for your wives, exactly as Christ did for the church—a love marked by giving, not getting. Christ's love makes the church whole. His words evoke her beauty. Everything he does and says is designed to bring the best out of her, dressing her in dazzling white silk, radiant with holiness. And that is how husbands ought to love their wives. They're really doing themselves a favor—since they're already "one" in marriage.

Just because you are not a wife in the "wedded bliss" sense of the word, don't disregard this passage of Scripture. It applies to all who are married to Christ through a relationship with Jesus. God uses the special union between man and wife to give us a glimpse of how important our bond is to him. He is our main man, savior, provider, protector, and best friend. "Everything he does and says is designed to bring the best out of her. . . ." God wants the best through us and for us, and so he has provided the way.

Soulful Solutions

One of the first duties of the new bride is to set up house. The same is true of your relationship with God. It's time to get your spiritual house in order. There are four basic steps you'll need to follow. We are going to rebuild who you are with God's plans for you in mind.

Step #1—Reorganize

Reorganize your priorities so they align with God's plan for your life. In order to do this you need to start thinking in terms of, "What would God want me to do or what would he want me to say?" This is a whole new approach to life. It's time to outgrow the "me first" attitude and change it to "God first." This won't be easy but with a little encouragement it becomes manageable. My advice to you (taken from Matthew 6:33–34) is to take it one day at a time, and rely on God's help.

Matthew 6:33–34 (MESSAGE)—Steep your life in God-reality, God-initiative, God-provisions. Don't worry about missing out. You'll find all your everyday human concerns will be met. Give your entire attention to what God is doing right now, and don't get worked up about what may or may not happen tomorrow. God will help you deal with whatever hard things come up when the time comes.

Step #2—Regroup

Peer pressure makes a huge impact on your life. Our friends play a major role in who we are and who we become as individuals. They affect how we act, what we wear, where we go, what we do, and what we say. They are highly influential in how we handle our lives, for the good or for the bad.

God's custom designed **bridal gown** fits every occasion.

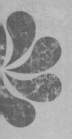

When a bride gets married, her friendships often change. She no longer has as much in common with the friends she had before she married, and she starts building new friendships. This same pattern holds true in your life as a Christian. Once you become the bride of Christ your interests, desires, and friends change too. This may sound like a bad thing at first, but it's a needed thing if your old friends had a negative impact on you.

The right friends make all the difference in the world. Are you hanging with people who influence you for the positive or for the negative? Take a candid look at the crowd you associate with and then determine if you need to regroup.

Proverbs 1:10 (MESSAGE)—Dear friend, if bad companions tempt you, don't go along with them.

Step #3—Rearrange

The next item on the agenda involves rearranging your schedule to accommodate quiet time alone with God. This is vital to your overall spiritual growth. The time we spend with God strengthens every part of us; mentally, physically, emotionally, and spiritually. Spending time regularly in prayer and Bible reading not only nurtures us as Christians but it also gives us direction for living according to God's plan for our lives. God leads and guides us through his Word, prayer, and the circumstances that surround us.

Mentally

Bible knowledge and prayer for discernment affect the way we think.

Romans 12:1–2 (MESSAGE)—So here's what I want you to do, God helping you: Take your everyday, ordinary life— your sleeping, eating, going-to-work, and walking-around life—and place it before God as an offering. Embracing what God does for you is the best thing you can do for him. Don't become so well adjusted to your culture that you fit into it without even thinking. Instead, fix your attention on God. You'll be changed from the inside out. Readily recognize what he wants from you, and quickly respond to it. Unlike the culture around you, always dragging you down to its level of immaturity, God brings the best out of you, develops well-formed maturity in you.

> Read one chapter of Proverbs every day. There are thirty-one chapters, which means you can **read it** in a month.

Physically

Bible application and prayer affect our habits. They help us make choices about what we will do with our bodies, including whether we'll be involved with drugs, alcohol, and premarital sex.

1 Corinthians 6:19–20 (MESSAGE)—Or didn't you realize that your body is a sacred place, the place of the Holy Spirit? Don't you see that you can't live however you please, squandering what God paid such a high price for? The physical part of you is not some piece of property belonging to the spiritual part of you. God owns the whole works. So let people see God in and through your body.

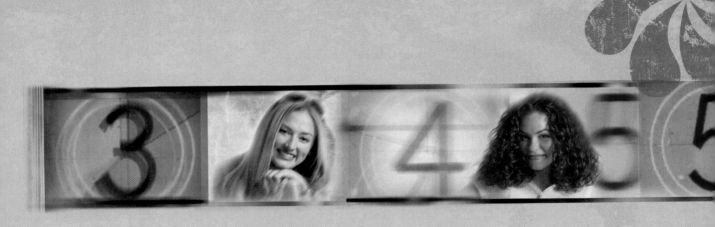

Emotionally

Bible understanding and prayer for self-control affect the way we react.

Proverbs 15:13,15 (MESSAGE)—A cheerful heart brings a smile to your face; a sad heart makes it hard to get through the day. A miserable heart means a miserable life; a cheerful heart fills the day with song.

Spiritually

Bible reading and prayer for insight increase our spiritual maturity.

Galatians 2:20 (MESSAGE)—I have been crucified with Christ. My ego is no longer central. It is no longer important that I appear righteous before you or have your good opinion, and I am no longer driven to impress God. Christ lives in me. The life you see me living is not "mine," but it is lived by faith in the Son of God, who loved me and gave himself for me. I am not going to go back on that.

God wants you to rely on him for everything from supplying the basics like underwear to providing you with money for college. Communication is key to developing this trust in the Lord. He desperately wants to communicate with you, but you must remember that communication lines work both ways; you get out of it what you put into it. If you only talk to God in church on Sundays, don't expect much out of the relationship. But if you rely on him day in and day out, your faith will grow with great expectation for what God is going to do next.

Step #4—Replenish

If steps one, two, and three sound a bit extreme, don't lose hope. Step four will help you find emotional strength and encouragement to press on with rebuilding your life.

Although this step is listed last it certainly is not least. You need to replenish your spirit on a regular basis by attending church with a local body of believers. Worship, Bible study, and prayer with like-minded individuals will further your spiritual walk, increase your faith, and reinforce your relationship with the Lord. Worshipping God gives you a spiritual high that you can only experience when you are glorifying him. Bible teaching by someone knowledgeable about the Word will give you insight into how the Bible applies directly to you. Praying over specific requests with other Christians motivates you to keep each other accountable before God.

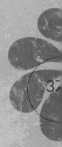

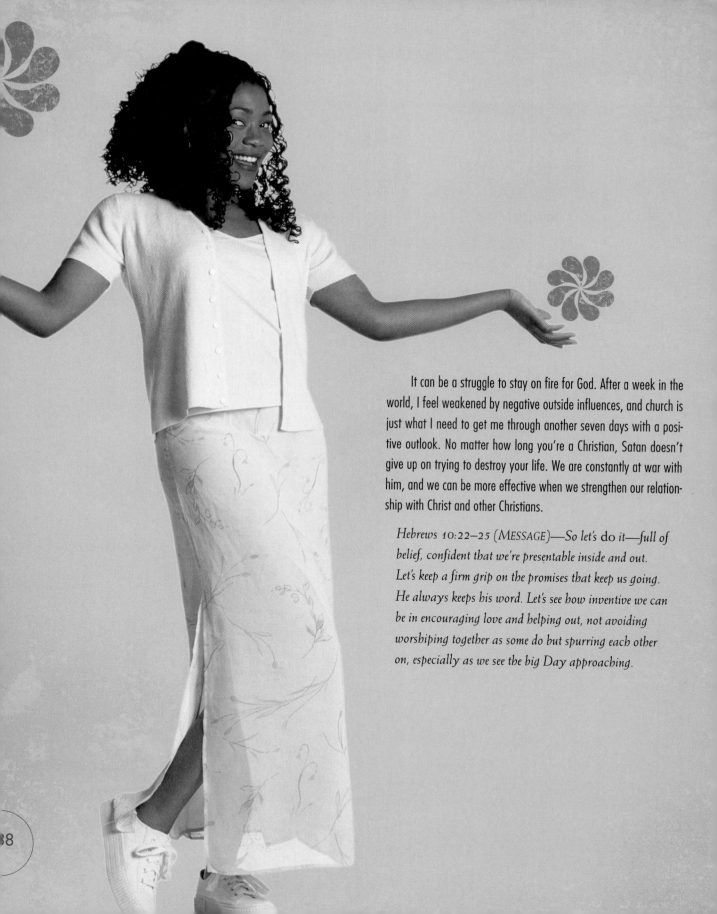

It can be a struggle to stay on fire for God. After a week in the world, I feel weakened by negative outside influences, and church is just what I need to get me through another seven days with a positive outlook. No matter how long you're a Christian, Satan doesn't give up on trying to destroy your life. We are constantly at war with him, and we can be more effective when we strengthen our relationship with Christ and other Christians.

Hebrews 10:22–25 (MESSAGE)—So let's do it—full of belief, confident that we're presentable inside and out. Let's keep a firm grip on the promises that keep us going. He always keeps his word. Let's see how inventive we can be in encouraging love and helping out, not avoiding worshiping together as some do but spurring each other on, especially as we see the big Day approaching.

The struggles you face each day are not actually against flesh and blood, as it may seem; they are against Satan and his dark spiritual forces. They create all of the havoc you are up against. It's like the movie Star Wars brought to life. You have the good guy, Luke Skywalker, fighting Darth Vader, who has joined forces with the dark side. It's an age-old story of good versus evil. Do you recall the most famous line of the movie? "May the force be with you." Luke was granted the power to win the battle, but he had to keep the faith. In fact he even had a special sword that helped him on his quest.

We can't live in the movies, but we can be like Luke Skywalker battling against the evil one. Our "force" is the Holy Spirit, and God enables us to conquer the dark side. Just as Luke Skywalker received training and a light saber to defeat the enemy, God furnishes us with the armor of God.

Ephesians 6:11–13—Put on the full armor of God so that you can take your stand against the devil's schemes. For our struggle is not against flesh and blood, but against the rulers, against the authorities, against the powers of this dark world and against the spiritual forces of evil in the heavenly realms.

In the chapters to follow we're going to look at each part of the armor. We'll learn about the defensive pieces and how they fit together to give us absolute protection. And we'll also look at the only offensive weapon: the sword. By the end of this book you will be outfitted from head to toe, fully equipped to conquer anything Satan dishes out.

✳ What This Means 2U

Every occasion calls for special clothing. And our spiritual lives are no different. Like a bride wearing her gown, ready to begin her marriage, we must dress for our journey. Fortunately for us, God knew what we were up against before the very foundation of the world and provided us with the perfect outfit to ensure stability in our relationship with him. He designed the armor of God to defeat outside influences that want to put our relationship with Jesus Christ on the rocks.

Ephesians 6:13—Therefore put on the full armor of God, so that when the day of evil comes, you may be able to stand your ground, and after you have done everything, to stand.

Super Models **rebuild** from the inside out

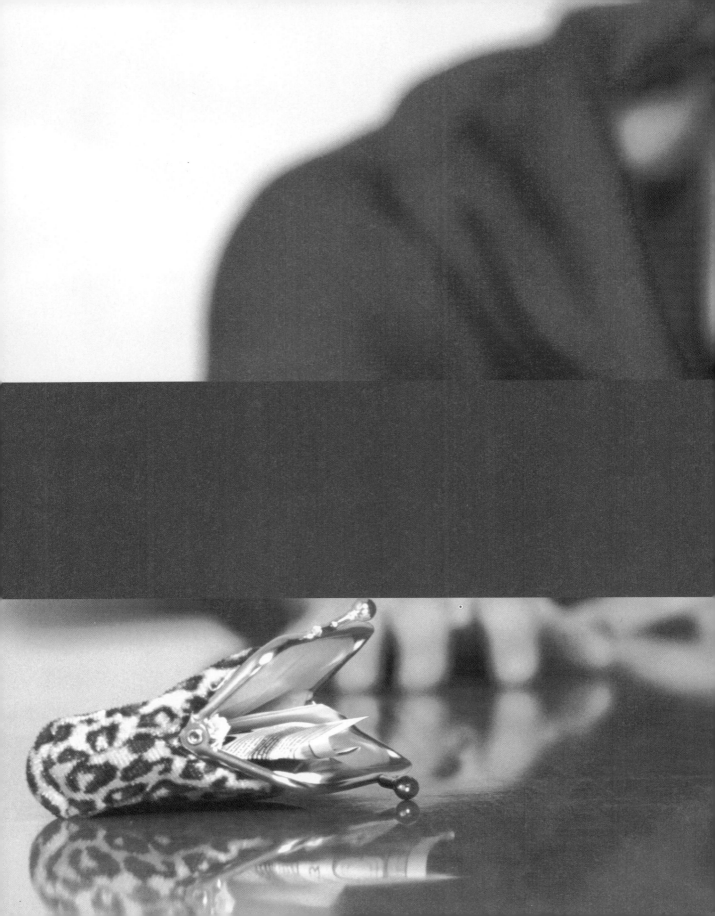

Accessorize, Accessorize, Accessorize

Part One—Belt It Up

After cleaning out your closets and rebuilding your wardrobe, you are ready to accessorize! Most women save accessorizing for last, but we're looking at the topic now so that we can accessorize what we already have on hand. Why start from scratch when a few updated fashion accessories can give an old wardrobe a new look for a lot less? ✻ Accessories often become "Afterthoughts," as one store puts it. Only after purchasing the shirt, pants, and shoes do we give any consideration to matching accessories. In fact, we rarely factor them into our clothing budget at all, making do with what we already have on hand. While this approach can work, it can also miss the target entirely. Why buy a cool shirt and the latest jeans and then neglect pulling the outfit together with the right accessories? Accessories can make your outfit hit a bull's-eye or miss the target altogether.

There are so many accessorizing possibilities that I hardly know where to begin. Of course, there are the basics: belts, bracelets, and necklaces. But what about barrettes, brooches, and bezels on watches? All of these can have a positive or negative effect on the way we look. Accessories complete our look; without them we are only partially put together.

As you make your shopping list, don't forget the extras that make everything you wear outstanding. Without the right accessories your new look won't be complete. In fact, some outfits can be accessorized in different ways to achieve a variety of looks. Don't believe me? Read on.

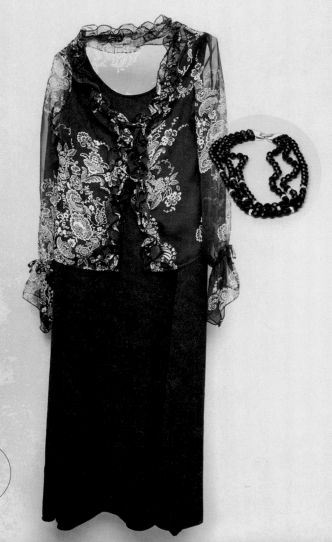

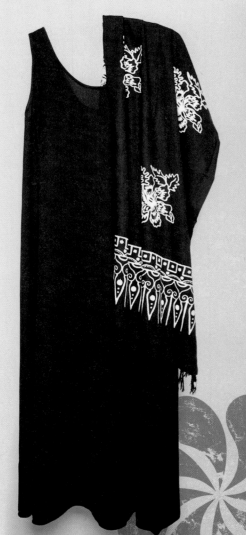

✳ Simple Solutions

I have an inexpensive basic black dress that I have owned for several years. It's yet to go out of style because I keep changing the accessories. I can dress it up for a semiformal evening out, or I can dress it down for casual occasions. For example, if my husband takes me out for a fancy dinner, I can add heels, a pearl necklace, and a scarf to give me a dressy look. For a picnic in the park, I'll give the dress a casual look by wearing simple sandals and no jewelry. The only thing required is a little creative ingenuity. Take a look at some of your own outfits. Can accessories be used to jazz them up or tone them down?

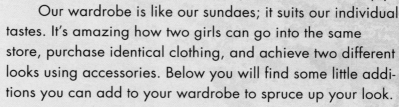

The answer to so many of your wardrobe worries can be solved with simple garnishing goodies. Getting outfitted is like eating ice cream. You can eat one scoop of plain old vanilla or you can dress it up a bit and have a sundae complete with hot fudge, caramel, whipped cream, and a cherry on top. Or maybe you prefer swirls of strawberry with crushed pineapple and chocolate chips; whatever suits your fancy, just create it and enjoy!

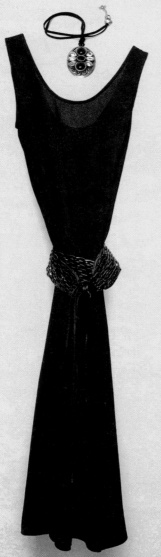

Our wardrobe is like our sundaes; it suits our individual tastes. It's amazing how two girls can go into the same store, purchase identical clothing, and achieve two different looks using accessories. Below you will find some little additions you can add to your wardrobe to spruce up your look.

Belts to Buckles

Everything from the width and color of your belt to the size and shape of your buckle can determine whether or not you're meeting current trends. There are so many accessories on the market I can hardly name them all: buttons, scarves, handbags, necklaces, earrings, bracelets, shoelaces, backpacks, hose, and hats. Of course, if that isn't enough then there are the fashion fads such as today's rub-on tattoos or the fifties' infamous poodle skirts. It seems like every generation has a "got to have it" gimmick. I advise that you don't go overboard on trendy items. Hot little doodads that are here today and gone tomorrow are not a wise wardrobe investment.

Be smart with your dollars; buy inexpensive accessories that look good. Savvy shopping saves money.

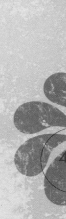

Size and Shape

Remember your size and shape as you pick out additions to your wardrobe. You want to wear your accessories; you don't want the accessories to wear you. If you have a small frame, avoid large accessories and if you have a larger frame, don't wear accessories that are too small. For example, petites shouldn't wear an extra-wide belt. Even if wide belts are in style, wearing a medium-width belt will accomplish the same look without being too overpowering. The same is true if you are full-figured. Wearing a narrow belt will go unnoticed and can actually make you look bigger by being ill proportioned. Keep these basic ideas in mind, and your accessories will always be well suited for you.

Hair

Many women overlook a major accessory—their hairstyle. How you fix your hair can make or break an outfit. Let's say that it's prom night and you're wearing a shimmering gown, dazzling jewelry, and snappy sandals but you have no plans for your hair. You've just ignored a major accessory. Healthy, great-looking hair is an asset to any wardrobe whether or not you accessorize it. Find a fashionable hairstyle by flipping through magazines and exploring your options. Once you find what you are looking for, take the picture with you to your hair appointment so the hairstylist can see exactly what you want. A picture is worth a thousand words when it comes to letting the stylist know how you'd like your hair to look. Also, remember to take any hair accessories you want added to your hairdo such as barrettes, combs, and flowers.

Spruce up clothing with lace, buttons, bows, glitter, beads, bangles, and anything else you can think of!

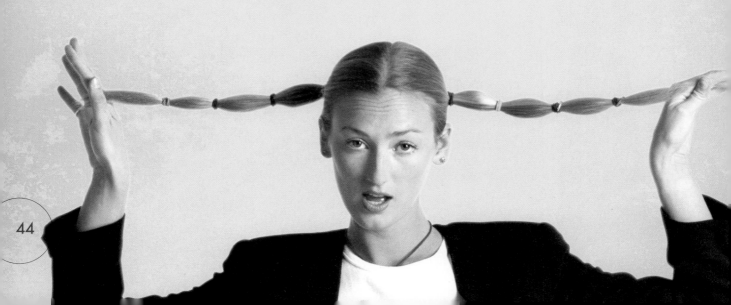

Gloss to Shadow

Consider your makeup as you accessorize your wardrobe. Do you need a makeover? When was the last time you evaluated your skin care and makeup routines? Healthy-looking skin and well-applied cosmetics create a stunning look. New lip glosses and eye shadows are two fashion accessories that change with every season. For just a few dollars you can give your face an updated look. For more information on this topic please read my book about beauty. You'll be glad you did!

Tips of Fingers to Tops of Toes

When was the last time you gave yourself a manicure or pedicure? Fixed-up fingernails and touched-up toenails are terrific ways to improve your image. With the countless colors of nail polish on the market you can match everything in your wardrobe. If that sounds like too much work, opt for neutral polish or a French manicure that will match it all without as much effort.

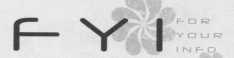

F Y I
FOR
YOUR
INFO

Name brands can be accessories when we want to project a certain image. If labels weren't so important, we wouldn't be spending so much money on them. But wearing name brands isn't everything, and it won't really change your life. The only life that will change is the designer's—he or she is getting rich off of your instinctive need to fit in. You are privileged if your parents can afford to keep you outfitted in name brand designers, but remember that not everyone is that lucky. What really matters isn't the labels you wear, but the way you treat others. Be sensitive to others who are less fortunate than you; put feelings before fashion.

Time Out
with Sammy

When I was in school Levi's were in vogue, and so it was my heart's desire to have that little tag hanging from my rear pocket; except I had one problem, my mother. She considered blue jeans of poor taste and refused to buy me any. I begged her until I finally came home from school one day to find a new pair of jeans on my bed. But they weren't Levi's, they were a generic name I had never heard of. I couldn't wear some off-name no one had ever heard of. They had to be Levi's or nothing.

The following weekend I went to a yard sale and found a pair of Levi jeans that were toddler size 4, but I bought them anyway. I took them home, removed the little orange tag, and sewed it onto the back pocket of my no-name jeans. Instant Levi's!

You're probably thinking, "How chintzy!" It might sound awful to you but it made me feel better. It just goes to show what drastic measures we'll stoop to in order to have the right trademark on our bottoms!

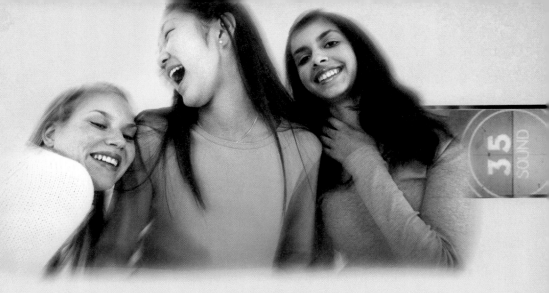

✳ What This Means 2U

Creative accessorizing is like getting a clothing makeover. I recently bought a cotton jacket off the clearance rack at Wal-Mart for only six dollars. It looked OK, but it needed a little something extra, so I changed the buttons and added shoulder pads. Now it looks like a million bucks!

Accessorizing can be the difference between average and outstanding. Fashionable accessories can bring last year's wardrobe up to date, enhance today's styles, and improve clothes that need a little extra help, all at a minimal cost. Accessorizing makes all the difference in the world when it comes to making a great fashion statement. While your target may be to look good, you can hit the bull's-eye by zeroing in on every detail. Accessories are key to a winning wardrobe.

Save **money** by giving your wardrobe a makeover.

❥Test It Out

Not sure what to do with last year's jeans? Try bringing them up to date with new accessories such as a belt, glitter, or fringe. Still not sure what to do with that tired old shirt? Spruce it up with cool buttons or a new necklace and earrings. Be creative! Accessories are just what you need to hook yourself up with a great new look for less. Take an inventory of your current accessories. Then use the form below to determine what you still need.

Renew

Do you have anything in your renew pile that still needs help? What about your closet or dresser drawers?

Item: Accessory idea:

Item: Accessory idea:

While making a list of what you need is helpful, it's often not enough. In some cases you might want to take the item with you to match it up with the accessories you want to add. You might need to try it on to match certain accessories such as belts, earrings, shoes, or scarves.

Part Two—Belt of Truth

Wow! So far we've learned how to have a relationship with God, rebuild our lives according to his plan, and recognize where our struggles come from. "For our struggle is not against flesh and blood, but against the spiritual forces of evil in heavenly realms" (Eph. 6:12). It is easier for Christians to fight in this spiritual battle when the master designer outfits us. Yes, there are clothes designed for every season and occasion, even spiritual combat. God has provided the perfect one-of-a-kind outfit that will never go out of style. It protects in all seasons of life and is perfectly suited for every occasion. This phenomenal fashion is known as the armor of God, a must-have in every Christian's wardrobe. ✳ You don't have to go shopping for this armor, and it's available right now for free. God provides directions in the Bible on just exactly how to put it all together, and it begins with an accessory. So let's head on over to God's accessory department and get measured for the first item on our armor list, the belt of truth.

There are several pieces of armor we're going to put on, and the very first piece is a critical accessory that holds the rest of the armor together. Without the belt of truth there is no breastplate of righteousness, shoes of peace, shield of faith, helmet of salvation, sword of the Spirit, or need of prayer. Everything hinges on truth, and not the world's version of truth, but God's version of Truth.

In this chapter you're going to learn how to identify right from wrong by putting everything you say and do to God's Truth test. This test works like a lie detector test—you can detect truth from fiction by hooking it up to the Word of God and comparing the answers against Scripture. This practice will keep you fastened in the belt of truth.

Operating off fact instead of fiction leads to a happy, healthy, helpful life in Christ—happy because there is contentment in applying truth, healthy because a truthful relationship benefits your overall well-being, and helpful because knowing the absolute truth gives you direction in every area of your life.

Satan often manipulates the truth to draw us away from God. That old devil is much more crafty than we give him credit for. That's why the Bible warns us about where our true struggles come from. Before we get dressed in the armor of God, we need to know what we're up against. After identifying the adversary, we need to devise a game plan to beat him at his own game. But before we're ready for the playing field we have to dress for the competition, and ours is a battle to outwit, outlast, and out-play Satan. Does it sound a little like *Survivor*? It's a game of sur-vival all right, but in this particular version, anyone who doesn't know the Lord is voted out, everyone who has accepted Christ will win, and you never have to go it alone because you have an alliance with God. So if you're ready, let the games begin.

The belt of **truth** is not measured by waist but by Word.

Soulful Solutions

Ephesians 6:14—Stand firm then, with the belt of truth buckled around your waist.

Stand firm for the truth according to God's purpose and plan. God's way is absolute Truth; Satan's way is adjusted truth. God's Truth is unchanging; Satan's truth changes every time you turn around, leaving you unsure about right and wrong. God's truth is spelled with a big *T*; Satan's truth is spelled with a little *t*; lowering the standard to tainted truth that leaves you confused and unable to make wise choices. Surviving Satan's tactics is dif-ficult but it can be done if you rely on God's Truth in everything you say and do. But it isn't always easy; Satan didn't earn the title "father of lies" for nothing.

Scripture It

Without the belt of truth tightly secured, you leave yourself vulnerable to the enemy's attack. Misunderstanding the truth will affect every area of your life. Below you will get an idea of what you're up against as we take the truth challenge—God's absolute Truth versus Satan's adjusted truth.

Emotional: Roller Coaster

Operating off your feelings will leave you on an emotional roller coaster. Absolute Truth is not based on how you feel about something; it's based on God. Satan would have you believe the alternative: "If it feels good, do it."

Situation: You want to go to a party (the kind where alcohol and drugs will be present) but you know your parents won't allow it, so what do you do?

> **God's Truth**—You are to obey your parents, so be willing to ask them for permission and then talk to them about why they made their decision. They aren't really party poopers; they just have your best interest in mind.

> **Satan's truth**—Ask your parents if you may spend the night at a friend's house and then go to the party with her. Satan's adjusted truth says, "What your parents don't know won't hurt them."

Emotionally, you feel confident that you can handle the party. You are not going to drink or do drugs, you only want to hang with your friends. But what happens when your friends are drinking and doing drugs? You've already loosened your belt if you lie to your parents, so chances are it's not secure enough to help you stand firm against peer pressure. Emotionally you feel the need to fit in, so saying, "no" isn't going to be easy when everyone around you is doing it.

Time Out
with Sammy

When I was a kid I had a lie detector machine that was powered by batteries. I used to amuse myself for hours by hooking unsuspecting victims up to my honesty device and watching them squirm until they couldn't take it anymore and ripped the prongs from their fingers. Of course, then they'd want to wire me up and ask me the questions. I'd willingly oblige because I knew how to make the little gizmo work on my behalf. You weren't supposed to move a muscle, but I knew how to move without getting caught. I'd firmly press my fingers into the surface that my hand was resting on until the little needle moved in the direction I wanted. Most of the time it worked, and rarely did I get caught at my own game.

Life is not all fun and games, but we can still manipulate the truth to correspond with our standards of morality. Here's a tough example. You may not like it, but it is based on God's Truth. The world's truth states that abortion is legal, but God's Truth says, "Thou shall not kill." Abortion is wrong because God is life and wants his followers to honor life. Truth measured against who God is (found in the Bible) will always be right even when the world states otherwise.

How are you wired? Do you base truth on what the world says or what the Word of God says? We can easily justify actions but remember, it takes action to justify the truth.

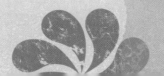

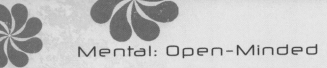

Mental: Open-Minded

Rational reasoning can cause you to deviate from God's absolute Truth. Satan wants us to believe that everyone must determine what is right and wrong in their own mind. In other words, if you **think** it's okay then it must be true.

Situation: You've received a take home test from your algebra teacher and the popular kids have invited you to their exclusive study group because they know you're smart. What do you do?

God's Truth—Say, "No, I can't make it tonight," even though you'd love to hang out with the popular kids. God's absolute Truth doesn't condone cheating, and you can't have honest relationships with people who use you.

Satan's truth—Satan will convince you to accept the invitation by adjusting the truth and justifying your actions. "It's just a take home test anyway, and if the teacher didn't want us to work together he would have had us take the test in class. We're not really cheating, we're just good friends helping each other out. I know all the answers anyway, so what I'm doing isn't wrong."

Mentally you are quite sure of yourself. And you try to determine what's right from your own vantage point of a situation. In your mind you didn't cheat, but what if the teacher's open-mindedness says otherwise? What if he decides to make an example out of you by failing you and allowing the rest of the group to retake the test in class? Sound fair? Not really. But when you leave everyone to decide truth in their own mind, anything is possible. That's why you must base your decisions on God's absolute Truth and avoid adjusting the truth to agree with your circumstances.

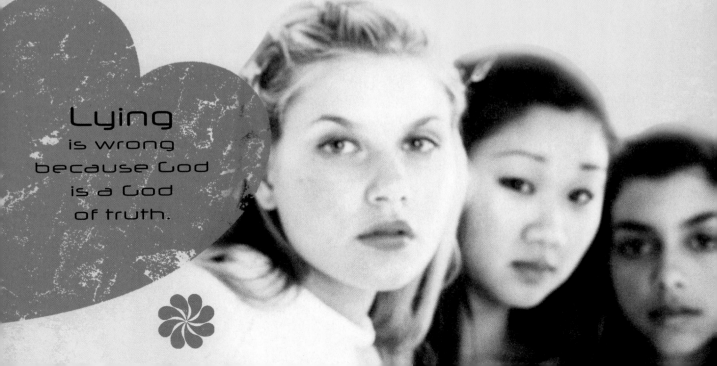

Lying is wrong because God is a God of truth.

Physical: Innate Need

Operating off physical desires can be harmful when you neglect God's absolute Truth. Innate needs can dictate your actions if you don't strap God's Truth around your waist.

Situation: You've been dating the same guy for three months, and he's putting the pressure on you to have sex. What's your response?

God's Truth—God states that sex outside of marriage is wrong. You can tell your boyfriend "no" and discover for yourself the truth of his feelings toward you. If he accepts your answer and agrees to wait then he really does care for you, but if he says, "so long," then you know his feelings were a lie from the start.

Satan's truth—Satan's adjusted truth says if you really care for your boyfriend you'll have sex. After all, you don't want to lose him, and if he doesn't get it from you, he'll get it from somebody else. If it's so wrong, why would school pass out condoms for protection?

Physically it's your body and you can do with it what you want. After all you plan on marrying him someday, so why wait? If God didn't expect you to have sex then why did he design the urge in the first place? All of these reasonings come from your physical urges, but God's absolute Truth still specifies that sexual relations of any kind should only take place within marriage. Sexual relationships outside of marriage will harm you emotionally, mentally, physically, and spiritually.

> **Cheating** is wrong because God is a God of integrity.

Spiritual: Value System

Are you at a place in your relationship with God where you rely on him for everything, or do you only call on him in emergencies? God's absolute Truth cares about every area of your life; no crisis is too big or too small for him to handle. He loves you so much that he gave his Son's life to save yours. But Satan hates you. He'll do anything, even adjusting the truth, to create in you a doubt of self-worth.

Situation: Your dad comes home and announces that his company is transferring him across country, which means that you will be leaving all your friends behind and changing schools. How do you handle it?

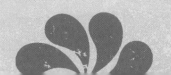

God's Truth—Disappointment will come naturally, but don't allow it to turn into depression. God's absolute Truth says, "I can do all things through Christ who strengthens me." It won't be easy on you or your family, but a good attitude will help.

Satan's truth—Satan's adjusted truth will tell you the exact opposite. You can't do it, you'll have no friends, and your parents are ruining your life. So run away. Satan will flash all kinds of horrible things through your mind so he can bring you down to the depths of despair.

If Satan can bring you down to where you no longer rely on God, then he's got you right where he wants you. I've known individuals who have sunk so low that they stopped praying because they had lost all hope. Satan jumps for joy when you are wallowing in misery. In times like these, when you lay all your spiritual values aside, he can tempt you with extreme anger, addictions, and even death.

These were some tricky truth scenarios. They may even sound like something you've encountered in your own life. Satan uses every pitfall he can to confuse you. If he can get you to doubt God's absolute Truth for even a second, then he can influence your morals and impact your actions. Don't give him the chance. Get your belt of truth on and keep it on.

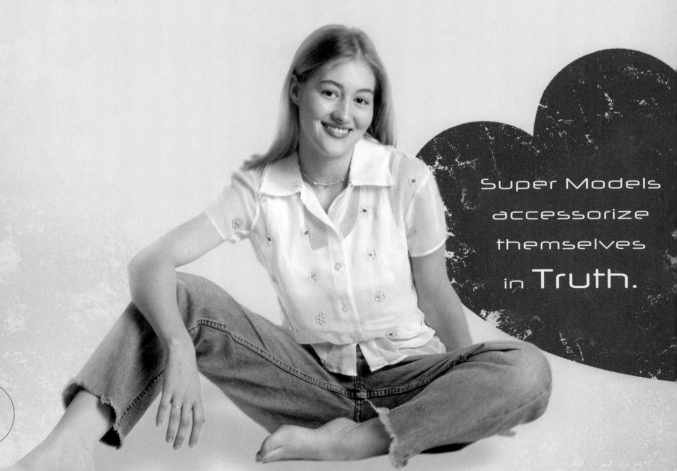

Super Models accessorize themselves in Truth.

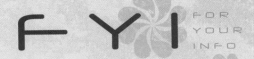

FYI
FOR YOUR INFO

Have you ever wondered if all this truth talk is for real? Well, guess what, people from all walks of life have wondered the same thing for years.

God is a God of absolute Truth and he expresses that truth in Scripture. But many people ask, "Is the Bible accurate and does it really hold true in today's society?" The answer to that question is, "Absolutely." There are many historical documents and archaeological discoveries that prove the Bible's accuracy. The biblical prophecies that were written thousands of years ago are being fulfilled even today. Still somewhat skeptical? Wondering how the Bible applies to you right here and now? I suggest prayer. God answers prayer. So ask God to show you how the Bible applies to you. What do you have to lose, besides your uncertainty?

Remember, apart from God there is no real truth. Those who don't know Christ personally have a difficult time understanding absolute Truth because they don't know the Truthmaker. They need a truth makeover, and you might be just the one to model the belt of truth.

✳ What This Means 2U

Without truth and trust, any relationship suffers hardships and undergoes adversity. God's way is absolute Truth, and in order to live a successful life you must be true to his leading. And because he loves you he's designed a visual aid, the armor of God, to help you dress for success.

Many scholars believe Paul was under house arrest when he wrote about the armor of God. He was probably guarded by Roman soldiers and may have even been chained to one. As he described the armor of God, Paul could just look up and jot down what he saw. To the people of Paul's time, seeing a Roman soldier walking about in his armor was customary, so Paul's detailed description gave them something to visually relate to. As we continue studying God's armor, I'd like to do the same for you. In the remaining chapters of this book I'll update the armor to resemble things we wear today.

❥ Test It Out

It's time to put on the truth belt and test it out. Wrap yourself in God's integrity and make absolute Truth a way of life. Remember, when you clothe yourself in God's belt of Truth, you're less likely to fall for Satan's adjusted truth.

Ephesians 6:14—Stand firm then, with the belt of truth buckled around your waist. . . .

Test everything you say or do against God's absolute Truth.

Read the Bible to discover God's absolute Truth.

Understand the difference between God's absolute Truth and Satan's adjusted truth so you can make wise choices.

Trust God to answer prayer.

Hold onto God's promises.

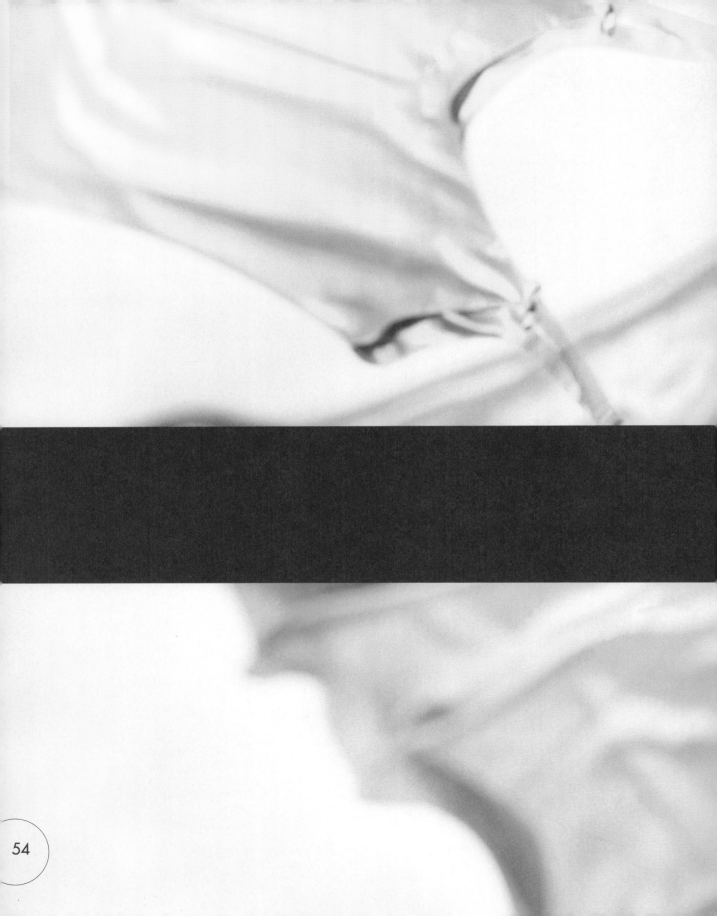

Under It All

Part One—Bottoms Up

t's time to talk about the bare essentials—your underwear. Not exactly the most popular subject, but one that needs review from the bottoms up. Buying bras and panties can be embarrassing; underwear is personal and most of us don't want to ask our mom or friends for an evaluation. We don't exactly try bras and panties on in the dressing room and then ask the salesperson, "Hey, how do these fit?" ✳ When you buy undergarments you're pretty much on your own. So where do you get the guidance you need to make

55

practical panty picks? The answer to that question and many more can be found right in this chapter. I'm going to give you panty advice, bra basics, and all the information you need to select great lingerie.

When I was younger, I was repeatedly warned that I didn't want to be caught in a car accident with dirty underwear on. I never understood that comment until I was in a serious automobile accident and the paramedic cut off my bra in order to save my life. Later, I kept thinking to myself, "It was clean, but I wish I'd been wearing a pretty, lacy bra that fit better." Those embarrassing thoughts made me determined to get a grip on undergarments. I didn't want to be caught with boring underwear again. And when I faced a similar situation a few years later, I felt more confident about the good-looking bra that was cut off.

Maybe you can't relate to having your underwear cut off, but what about the girls' locker room? I remember feeling self-conscious about what I was wearing underneath my clothes as I dressed for P.E. class. Let's face it; girls naturally compare themselves to other girls. We want to be accepted for who we are and what we wear—right down to our bra and panties. But how can we be sure that we're wearing the right thing? This can be an embarrassing topic, but I'm going to give you the details about size, shape, and style so you don't feel inhibited by your unmentionables anymore.

Getting dressed from the bottom up requires finding the right size for your shape and a style that flatters your figure. When you understand the needs of your body, you'll look and feel your best knowing that your wardrobe works for you—from the inside out.

✳ Simple Solutions

There are three S's to remember when shopping for lingerie: size, shape, and style.

Size—How to Measure Up

The most common mistake made when purchasing undergarments is choosing the wrong size. Many girls simply wear the wrong size bra and panties. To avoid sizing mishaps follow the steps below to select perfectly sized underwear.

Bra Size Step #1

Use a seamstress's measuring tape to measure around your rib cage just beneath your breasts. Be careful to keep the tape measure smooth and taut to get a precise measurement.

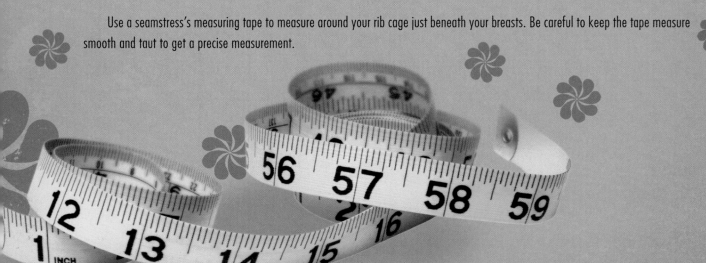

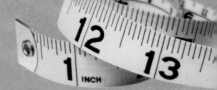

Bra Size Step #2

Add 5 inches (to an odd number) or 6 inches (to an even number) to your measurement in order to obtain your band size. For example, I measure at 29 inches, so I add 5 inches to get a 34-inch band size.

Record your equation here:

_____ (step 1 measurement) + _____ (5 or 6 inches) = _____ band size

Note: Band sizes only run in even numbers; thus the reason you must add 5 or 6 inches accordingly. On a bra with more than one latch, the exact measurement is found when you fasten the middle hooks.

Bra Size Step #3

Measure all the way around your chest at the fullest point of your bustline. To get a perfectly balanced measurement, hold the tape measure straight without making it so tight that your breasts smoosh together.

Record the measurement here: _____ inches

Time Out
with Sammy

Do you remember your first bra? I sure do. My mom used to play Bunco—a game where gabby women got together to roll dice for prizes. I never cared much about the game until the Bunco Christmas party during my fourth-grade year. My mother was hosting that year's party, and I was thrilled because my mom had promised that I could open a present during their annual gift exchange! I could hardly wait.

Eventually, the ladies finished the game, announced the winner, had their refreshments, and were ready to swap gifts. My mom called me to the center of the room and handed me a festively wrapped package. I love presents and the fact that I was the center of attention only added to my excitement—until I unwrapped the box and pulled out what was inside. It was a green and white-striped bra and panty set. I was horrified! I couldn't shove it back into the box fast enough as I raced out of the room. But it was too late; the ladies had already seen the gift and were laughing unmercifully. I could have died right there on the spot.

It was nearly a year before I worked up the courage to actually wear the bra, and when I finally did put it on, I kept it as my own little secret to avoid further teasing. But I didn't exactly know how to adjust the straps, and the fact that it was called a *training* bra made me wonder what it was training and how it was going to do it. My questions went unanswered because I wasn't about to suffer any further humiliation by discussing them with anyone.

What about you; do you have any lingering lingerie questions? Well don't despair; I'm here to help.

Bra Size Step #4

The difference between the breast measurement in step 3 and the band measurement in step 2 determines your cup size. For example, the measurement around the fullest point of my breast is 36 inches, and my band size is 34 inches—a difference of 2 inches. That makes my cup size a B, and my bra size a 34B.

Record your equation here:
_____ (step 3 breast size) - _____ (step 2 band size) = _____" difference

Each inch of difference is equal to one cup size:
  less than 1 inch = AA cup
  1 inch   = A cup
  2 inches = B cup
  3 inches = C cup
  4 inches = D cup
  5 inches = DD cup

Record your cup size here: _____

Note: Even though this method of measurement is quite dependable, I recommend you try at least three bra sizes on in order to get the perfect fit. For example, I measure as a 34B, so when I shop for a bra, I try it on in 34B, an up size of 36A, and a down size of 32C. Bra shopping is like jean shopping; you don't always wear the exact same size. Always try it on before buying.

Panties Size

Finding the perfect-sized panties is really quite simple. They usually run the same as your pant size. For example, if your jeans are a size 9, your panties will also be a size 9. When panties are made of a fabric that will shrink, such as cotton, you might want to purchase one size bigger to allow for shrinkage. Sometimes, underwear is sold in sizes small, medium, and large. These sizes are usually based on the size list below, but always check the back of the panty package for a size chart to be sure.

  Small (sizes 3–5)
  Medium (sizes 7–9)
  Large (sizes 11–13)

Shape with Style

Body shape will affect the style of underwear you choose, although panties are often picked based on personal preference rather than how they benefit your figure. I'm going to give you advice on how to shape up your body type with different styles of undergarments.

What is your body type?

- Pear Shape
- Rectangular Shape
- Apple Shape
- Hourglass Shape
- Wedge Shape

Pear Shape: You'll want to bring balance between your top and your bottom. I suggest a fully padded bra or a partially padded gel bra, lifting your breasts to create fullness on top. Use seamless control panties to minimize your lower half.

Rectangular Shape: You'll want to create natural-looking curves by enhancing your bustline. A push-up bra can be just the boost you need to enhance your figure without making it look ill-proportioned on top. For the bottom, bikini or low rise briefs will soften your angular shape.

Apple Shape: Apple-shaped gals are usually well-endowed. If this is true for you, then you should wear a bra that offers full coverage, which includes the area beneath your armpits. I recommend full-figured (control) panties that fit well and don't ride up.

Hourglass Shape: You'll need an under-wire lift or a full-coverage bra that will support the natural shape of your breasts without diminishing your natural curves. For panties, try seamless tummy control if this is a problem area.

Wedge Shape: If you have a wedge-shaped figure, you want to create softness and enhance the visual curve of the bustline by wearing a shaper or push-up bra. For underwear, try a pair of the comfy boy shorts.

Don't dress to get **attention** you really don't want.

59

FYI
FOR YOUR INFO

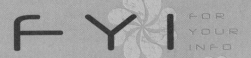

While finding the right underwear is often based on size, shape, and style, there is another "S" word that helps us make wardrobe decisions.

Self-Respect

Respecting yourself and others by the way you dress will improve your look as well as your outlook on life.

Undergarments used to be the cheapest part of your wardrobe, but I recently looked at a set of underwear that cost the same as the jeans I was wearing. At those prices, I figured I'd have to start wearing them outside my clothes so I could show them off. Maybe the cost is why today's styles are so revealing! Today, many girls throw modesty out the window by revealing their underwear (and more) by the way they dress.

Modesty is a serious issue, although we often view it as a lighthearted subject. Do you respect yourself in the way you dress? If you don't present yourself with class and dignity, don't expect others to treat you that way either, especially guys. They'll only respect you as much as you respect yourself.

Every girl's goal is to look good, but the question is how good? You can look good by dressing modestly, or you can be *looking good* by dressing sexy. Guys are visually stimulated, and when you dress sexy, you are tempting them to act inappropriately—toward you and even toward other girls.

The definition of sexy: sexually stimulating

I'm troubled by how many girls dress sexy without understanding what that entails. Dressing sexy means that you want to *provoke sexual stimulation*. And what happens when you stimulate guys? They want sex! In fact, I believe that revealing clothing has contributed to the rise of date rape. Dressing sexy leads to sex—both willingly and forcefully.

I'm not condoning a guy's terrible actions in date rape; I simply want you to understand how you could unintentionally provoke it by the way you dress. It's important to realize that clothing makes a statement. What do your clothes say about you? Are they revealing? Are they tight and form fitting? Can you see your underwear? Are your skirt and shorts too short or is your top low cut? You need to ask these important questions as you get dressed. Remember, when you respect yourself, others will respect you too.

What This Means 2U The perfect size, shape, and style of underwear will not only enhance your figure, it will also improve the fit of your clothes. No more puckered shirts from misfit bras and no more panty lines from poorly fitting panties. Even though you don't see undergarments, you'll notice immediately how wearing the right ones positively affects your entire wardrobe. You may think it doesn't matter what you wear beneath your clothes, but wearing the right lingerie makes all the difference in the world.

Test It Out

It's time to grab the tape measure and get started. How do your bras measure up? Are you wearing the right size and style for your shape? Look through a catalog or browse the lingerie department at your local store to discover just how many different types of bras and underwear are available, and then start trying them on.

It's safe to try on bras in the store, but panties are a different story. Some panties have built-in panty liners, but it's still not sanitary to try them on against your bare skin. I recommend that you take a pair of spandex shorts with you to wear while trying on panties or swimsuits. You'll get a good idea of how they fit without allowing them to make contact with your vaginal area. And remember; once you buy and take them home, be sure to wash them before you wear them.

Use the form below to help you shop and fill in where your wardrobe is lacking.

Bra Size

What size bra do you wear (see page 58)?

What is the equivalent up size?

What is the equivalent down size?

Do you need a new bra? If so what type and what color?

      Type:

      Color:

      Type:

      Color:

Panty Size

What size panties do you wear? (same as your pants size)

Do you need underwear? If so what type and what colors?

      Type:

      Colors:

      Type:

      Colors:

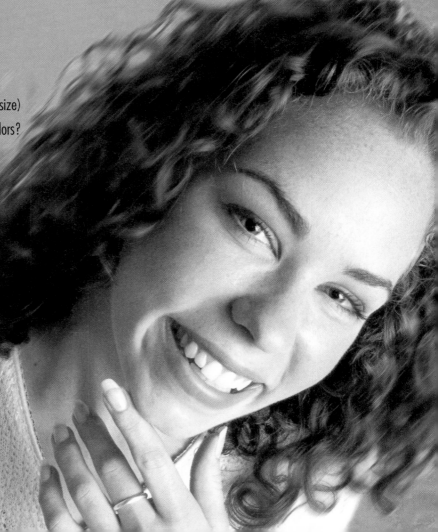

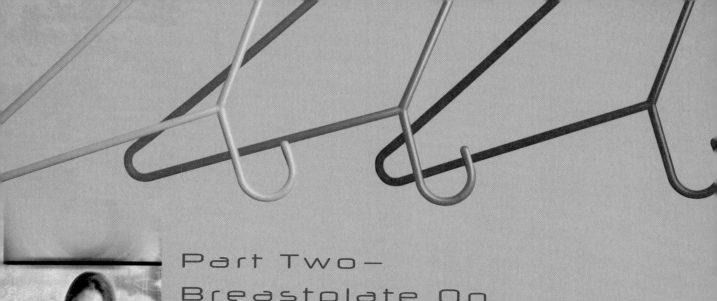

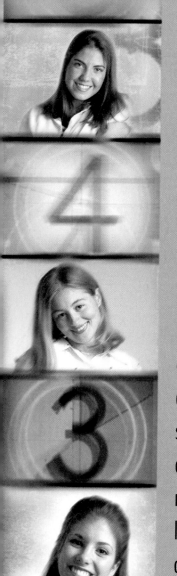

Part Two—
Breastplate On

With the belt of truth securely fastened around your waist, it's time to attach the breastplate of righteousness. The breastplate of righteousness serves as a bare essential, enabling you to resist the enemy's attack. It's similar to a bulletproof vest that protects your heart from injury or death. But if you want it to be effective, you must keep it securely in place at all times. Even a cop who is off duty needs to wear the vest to ensure his or her continual safety. Statistics show that a calculating enemy is more likely to strike when a cop's guard is down. Bottom line, it's never safe to be caught without your armor. ✳ We're going to examine several ways to keep our breastplate secure so it protects us, even when we're unaware of enemy attack. The devil is crafty, and he's just waiting to catch you off duty so he can do a number on you. Like an off-duty cop, you can leave your post, but don't leave yourself unprotected. Put on the breastplate of righteousness and attach it to the belt of truth to protect the heart of your character.

The heart of your character isn't based only on the moral standards you display before others. Sound character is shown by the choices you make, even when no one is watching you. Sometimes it's easier to make the right choices when you have an audience of teachers or parents. But when you're alone with your peers, or by yourself, doing the right thing gets tougher.

For example, what do you do if a salesclerk gives you the wrong change? She was supposed to give you $14.23 but instead of a ten, she accidentally pulled out a twenty and gave you $24.23. What should you do? A person suited up in the breastplate of righteousness displays moral character and gives back the twenty in exchange for the proper change.

Putting on the breastplate of righteousness will help you handle these situations, as well as many others that you will face in life.

Ephesians 6:14—Stand firm then, with the belt of truth buckled around your waist, with the breastplate of righteousness in place.

In order to combat Satan and his evil forces you must be fully equipped. In chapter 3 we applied the belt of truth, and now we need to add the breastplate of righteousness. We must protect our heart and emotions, which affect our thoughts and control our actions. God's righteousness is the breastplate that will help you stand firm when your character is under attack. So, if you're ready, let's size it, shape it, and style it for a fit that's just right.

Soulful Solutions

Have you ever noticed that the enemy knows exactly where you are most vulnerable? He plots and charts our every move so he knows where our weaknesses lie. It's like we are being stalked. Although invisible to the naked eye, Satan's dark forces surround us, seizing any opportunity to make us mess up.

Although we have different weaknesses, we can each find strength in applying the breastplate of righteousness. It won't stop Satan's attacks, but it will help us withstand them. So let's get sized for a custom fit.

Size—How to Measure Up

God's righteousness is a one-size-fits-all breastplate. Whether or not it works depends on the way you apply it. If you are one of those people who thinks their breastplate doesn't quite measure up, read on so you can receive a tailored fit.

Scripture Step #1

Size up what the Word of God says. Reading the Bible will give you insight for everyday living.

Scripture Step #2

Start a Bible study; either get involved with a group study or do one on your own. This will help you learn the Word and how it applies directly to you.

> The breastplate of righteousness **shapes** and supports the character of God within us.

Scripture Step #3

Try the 5/R method of verse study: Read, WRite, Rediscover, Redefine, and Reinforce. Select a topic and then use a concordance to jot down verses pertaining to that topic. (1) *Read* the verse, (2) *write* the verse, (3) *rediscover* the same verse in other Bible translations, (4) *redefine* the verse so that it applies to you personally, and (5) *reinforce* it with prayer.

Scripture Step #4

Devote the Word of God to memory. I can't begin to tell you how beneficial this is in times of trouble. It's amazing how a verse that I memorized years ago will come to mind exactly when I need it. God's Word is faithful and true.

1 Thessalonians 5:17 (MESSAGE)—Pray all the time.

Prayer

Prayer is vital when it comes to securing and maintaining the armor of God. The verse above tells us to keep the lines of communication open. God is available to listen 24/7, so pray whenever or wherever you need to. God is there. It doesn't matter if you have a small, medium, or large problem, he's waiting to hear from you.

Scripture It

Shape and Style

When you allow God to shape and mold your life in his righteousness, your life will meet with his approval.

2 Timothy 2:15—Do your best to present yourself to God as one approved, a workman who does not need to be ashamed and who correctly handles the word of truth.

Our lives will be shaped by trials and adversity. I once heard it said: "Life is 10 percent what happens to us and 90 percent how we react to it." This is true. Your attitude is a choice, and it's key to successful living. When you shape your attitude to align with God's Word and support it with prayer, God's righteousness will become more evident in how you react.

Not every difficult ordeal that you face will be a direct result of something that you've said or done. We're often put into situations we never asked for, yet we're expected to handle them in a positive manner. On the outside it may seem unfair that you should handle these situations with an optimistic attitude. But when you take a look at how it affects your inside, you'll notice immediately why this is the right thing to do.

Proverbs 23:7 (NKJV)—For as he thinks in his heart, so is he.

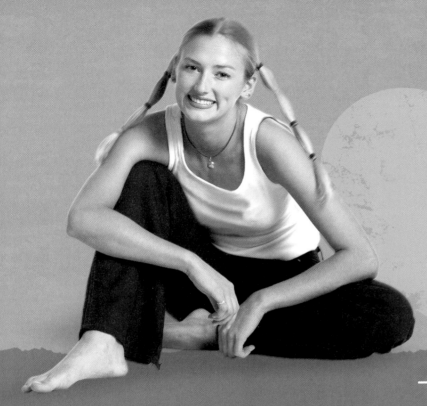

ABILITY
TO
TOLERATE
IMPOSING
TRIALS
UTILIZING
DIVINE
EXPRESSION

Time Out
with Tammy

I used to think I couldn't talk to God unless it was pertaining to something major, like a debilitating illness or financial destitution. It seemed like all the prayers in church were about some grandiose problem. I had never dreamed that God was interested in communicating with me about nothing in particular.

One time I was devastated because I didn't make the cheerleading squad. I felt like I didn't have a friend in the world. You see, it was the student body that was responsible for picking the cheerleaders, and when I didn't get picked I didn't feel very well liked. When they announced the results over the loudspeaker at school I wanted to crawl under a desk and hide, but instead I had to muster up the energy to face the bus ride home.

When I finally got home I ran into my room and burst into tears. I remember blubbering to God, "Why didn't you let me get picked?" And then I realized I hadn't ever asked for his help. For some reason I thought praying to God about something for myself would make him mad or disappointed with me. I didn't understand how much he really cared about every single detail in my life, right down to cheering for the guys' football and basketball teams.

With the next day of school just hours away, I prayed and asked God to end feelings of jealousy about my best friend who had made the cheerleading squad. I wanted to be happy for her no matter how much I grimaced at the thought. And you know what? It worked. I was able to withstand the negative comments made toward me without resentment and I could celebrate with my girlfriend over her victory. One of the teachers even recommended that I try out for the pom-pom squad, and guess what? This time I prayed and made it!

Prayer changes things!

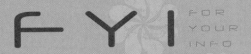

FYI
FOR YOUR INFO

Although you may be reading the Bible consistently, praying constantly, and continually checking your attitude, there's still one major issue to consider.

Self-Esteem

Do you hold yourself in high esteem or do you put yourself down? A poor self-image holds you back from becoming all that God desires you to be. Satan uses this to break down our defenses more than anything else. If he can cause us to doubt our self-worth, then he can cast a shadow of doubt in other areas of our life too, even our perception of right and wrong. The next time you start to feel worthless, remember these three important facts:

Important Fact #1

God loves you. 1 John 4:10—This is love: not that we loved God, but that he loved us and sent his Son as an atoning sacrifice for our sins.

Important Fact #2

God values you so much that he gave the life of his Son to save your life. John 3:16—For God so loved the world that he gave his one and only Son, that whoever believes in him shall not perish but have eternal life.

Important Fact #3

You are of great value. 1 Corinthians 6:20 (NKJV)—For you were bought at a price; therefore glorify God in your body and in your spirit, which are God's.

The value of something is driven by what someone will pay for it. Value isn't determined by a price tag unless the item is actually purchased for that amount. So what is the highest price that can be paid for something? What is the greatest gift and how much does it cost?

John 15:13 (NKJV)—Greater love has no one than this, than to lay down one's life for his friends.

❋ What This Means 2U
Understanding and utilizing the breastplate of righteousness will make all the difference in the world as you approach the trials of life. Although it acts like an invisible shield, you'll see the positive effect it has on your attitude. Protecting your heart, the seat of your emotions, through Bible study and prayer will shape your life into something beautiful from the inside out.

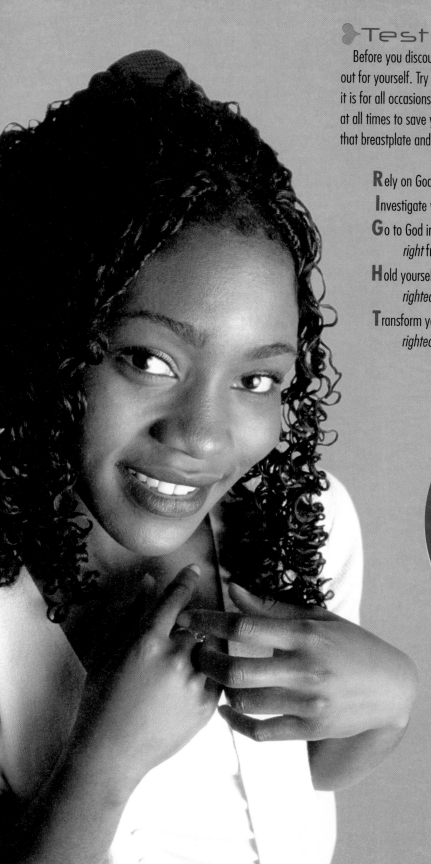

❥Test It Out

Before you discount the importance of the breastplate, test it out for yourself. Try it on for thirty days and see just how fitting it is for all occasions. Like a bulletproof vest, it has to be worn at all times to save you from enemy attack. So keep wearing that breastplate and choosing what is right:

Rely on God's *righteousness* to mold your character.

Investigate what the Bible says about *righteousness.*

Go to God in prayer and ask him to help you discern *right* from wrong.

Hold yourself in the highest esteem. God in his *righteousness* does.

Transform your attitude so it's in check with God's *righteousness.*

Super Models **guard** their hearts with righteousness.

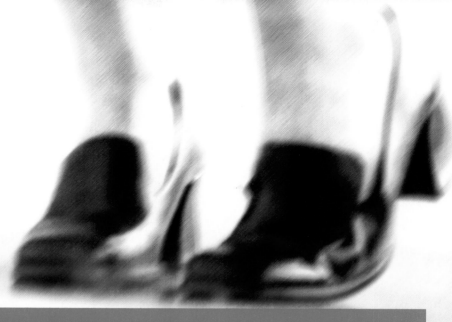

fancy footwear

Part One— Shoes for All Occasions

One pair won't do,
When it comes to a shoe.
Two pairs are nice,
But you better think thrice.
Four pairs are square,
Buy five if you dare.
Six pairs are great,
So why not seven or eight!
Nine, now that is enough,
No, ten, I need some in buff.
Eleven, twelve, and thirteen times four,
Holy Cow! I still want more.
Shoes, shoes are beautiful things,
A girl's best friends like diamonds in rings.

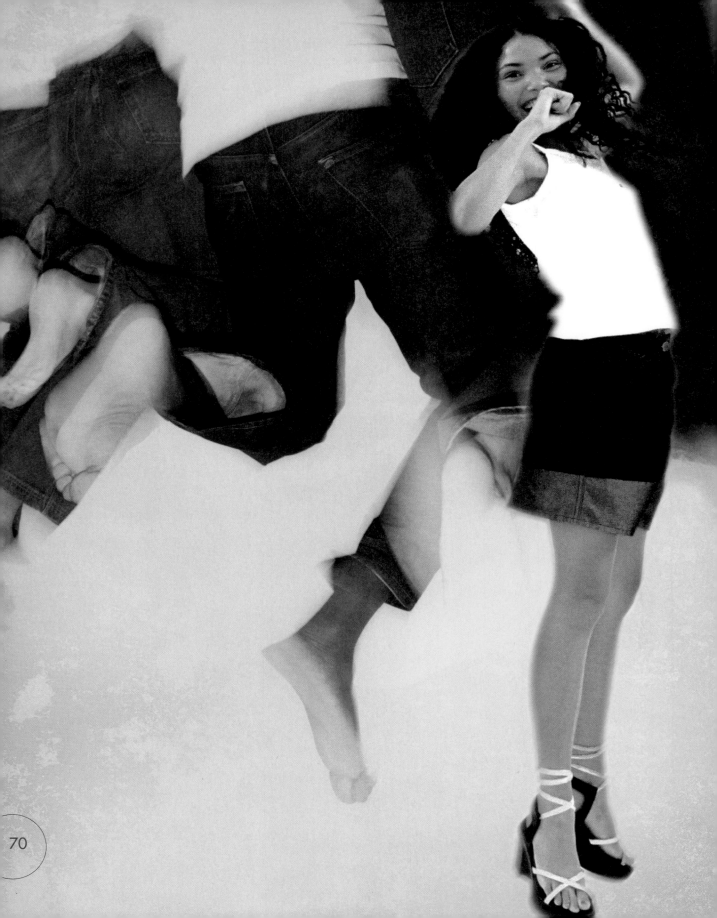

Can we ever have enough shoes? It seems as though every time I promise not to buy another pair, I find some cute, on sale, must-have shoes that are beckoning me to take them home. Yep, you guessed it, I'm a shoe-a-holic. I love shoes! ✳ Casual, dressy, athletic, or formal—shoes come in styles for every occasion. So we're going to spend this chapter talking about those glorious items we wear at the end of our ankles. Get cozy with your bunny slippers on and let's hop right in!

Remember the fairy tale about Cinderella? Did you breathe a sigh of relief when the prince slid the glass slipper onto Cinderella's little foot? It was a perfect match—and they lived happily ever after. There probably isn't a girl alive who hasn't wished for a fairy godmother, someone to wave a magic wand and create the perfect dress, hair, and shoes for them. We'd like to be whisked away by a white limo to the prom of our dreams—where we can dance with Prince Charming all night. In real life though, we often feel like the Cinderella who loses her dream when the clock strikes midnight. But don't worry, you know how the story ends—the shoe saves the day!

Although we can't live in a fairy tale, the Cinderella ending can hold true in real life. Perfect-sized shoes save the day, lending comfort and protection to our feet and accessorizing our wardrobe. And when you slide your aching feet into a soft pair of slippers after a grueling day of school, you'll relax and say, "Ahhh . . . they lived happily ever after."

If the Shoe Fits

My friend Rose always says, "If the shoe fits, buy it!" But before you go shoe shopping, there are a few things you need to know.

Simple Solutions

I once talked to an orthopedic surgeon who told me that many foot problems are due to people wearing the wrong size shoes—and females are the biggest offenders. I'm guilty of this very thing. I'll come across a pair of shoes on the clearance rack that are a half size too small, but I buy them anyway, thinking I'll stretch them out. This doesn't work very often, and my feet are miserable during the whole process. I often end up tossing the shoes. Take advice from the doctor and me, save yourself misery and money by following these two steps to happier, healthier feet.

Shoes **support** our arches as well as fashion.

Step #1—Size It Up

Take the guesswork out of shoe sizing by having a professional measure your foot. This free service is offered in the shoe department of most major retail stores, whether or not you purchase shoes. Make sure you have both feet measured because it is common to have one foot larger than the other. When this happens, you need to buy shoes based on the size of the larger foot.

Step #2—Try It On for Size

Now that you know what size you wear, try both shoes on for size. Don't assume that if you wear a size 9 every size 9 shoe will fit. To get a precise fit, put both shoes on and walk around in them. If they are athletic shoes, try moving in them as you would in the sport you are participating in. For example, if you are buying basketball shoes, try jumping, or if you are buying soccer shoes, then maneuver and kick.

The right-sized shoes are extremely important for everything from walking around school to playing in Saturday's game. Miserable, aching feet will negatively affect your mood, but when your feet are comfortable, you can focus on important things like your classes or the big game.

> Before you have your feet sized, make sure they are clean and odor free. If you have trouble with **stinky feet,** use a mint foot scrub and a liquid foot powder.

PICTURE IT

Shoes Help Outfit Every Style

Nothing says sensational style more than the appropriate pair of shoes. Shoes add class to almost any outfit. Are you going to the beach in a cute new swimsuit? Why not add an adorable pair of beaded flip-flops to match?

Shoes will either finish your outfit or leave you looking like something is missing. They come in a wide variety of styles and colors that are sure to upgrade any wardrobe. And the right shoe can make a big statement. So what kind of shoes are you wearing?

Below I've listed a variety of shoes to give you an idea of the various types on the market. Use this list to inventory your own shoe collection, noting which styles and colors you already have and which ones you'd like to add. Although the names may change the styles remain basically the same as fashion repeats itself every few years.

Brilliant Boots
Loafing Loafers
Happy Heels
Perky Platforms
Fabulous Flip-Flops
Super Sandals
Striking Slingbacks
Marvelous Mules
Snug Slippers
Sassy Stilettos
Pretty Pumps
Wonderful Wedges
Fancy Flats
Savvy Slip-Ons
Slick Saddle Shoes
Magnificent Mary
    Janes/Ballets
All-Star Athletics

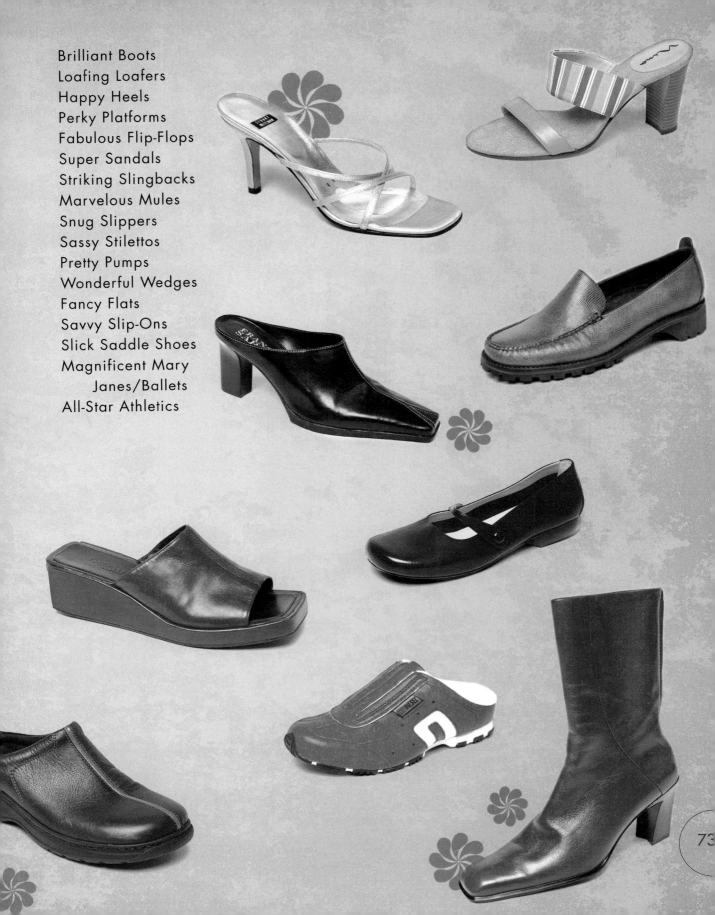

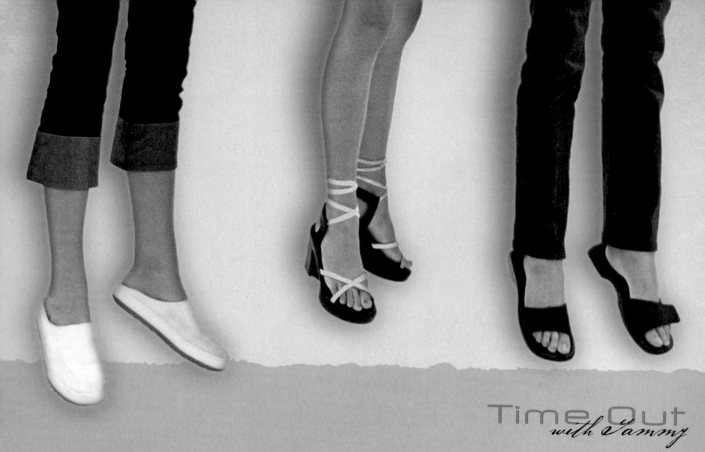

One year, a couple of my girlfriends took me to *The Price Is Right* to celebrate my birthday. I spent days planning what I would wear to the game show. I had an attractive dress but I needed some cute shoes to match. Two days before the event I found an adorable pair of narrow-toed flats adorned with puffy bows made of white tulle. Believe it or not, this really was in style back then! The morning of my birthday, I felt self-assured in the way I was put together, and we set off to seize the day.

One perk of being in *The Price Is Right* audience is that you might get chosen as a contestant. Hours before taping begins, everyone gathers outside the stage doors, hoping that the producers will select them as a contestant—one of the lucky few who get to play for cash and prizes. Just before it was my turn to be interviewed, I got nervous and ran to the ladies' room for a quick mirror check. Makeup, hair, lipstick—all were in order as I ran off to the audition.

I greeted the producers with a friendly smile and a firm handshake and confidently awaited their questions. The first thing they asked me was not, "What is your name and what are your hobbies?" but "Do you always wear toilet paper on your shoes?" At first I thought they were referring to my puffy shoe bows, but then I looked down at my feet and was horrified to see a long streamer of toilet paper trailing behind my left foot. I quickly regained my composure and replied, "Why yes, I thought it matched my shoes so well that I brought it with me just in case one of my bows fell off." They chuckled and then yelled, "Next!"

Well, even though I made a spectacle of myself, I still didn't get selected to participate on stage. But I did learn two things. First, learn to laugh at yourself, and second, when you go to the ladies' room, check your makeup, hair, lips, and *shoes!*

There is a basic rule to follow as you pick shoes for skirted outfits: the shorter the dress, the shorter the heel. The following guidelines will help you match the height of your shoes to your dress length so your legs look proportionally balanced.

Let's start from the top and work our way down.

Miniskirts look best with flat shoes such as loafers, slip-ons, or sandals.

Skirts or dresses that come near the kneecap look best with 1- or 2-inch heels such as mules, wedges, and pumps.

Mid-calf dresses or skirts look best with 1- or 2-inch heels such as platforms, sling backs, pumps, or knee-high boots. Stilettos are a great option for evening wear.

Ankle length skirts or dresses look great with a medium to high heel, platform or wedge.

Formal wear should always be graced with medium to high-heeled shoes unless you're trying to be shorter than your date. In that case, a pair of flats are fitting for the occasion.

✳ What This Means 2U
Good shoes are not just the right style, color, or name brand; they also fit your feet well. It's easy to think that it doesn't matter what shoes feel like as long as they look good, but that notion can mess up your feet. Aching feet make life agonizing. And when our feet are unhappy, even those special occasions like the prom are less enjoyable.

Remember, expensive shoes are not always good shoes. I once bought a pricey pair of brand-named walking shoes that did more damage than good. I've also bought cheap knock-offs that were wonderfully comfortable.

To **elongate** your legs (and make you look taller and thinner) wear shoes and hose that are the same color as your pants or skirt.

❧Test It Out

As you go through your closet and decide which shoes to keep and which ones to get rid of, check the size, try them on, and then walk around to determine how they feel and fit. Prioritize your shoe needs. For everyday wear, begin with a pair of basic black or brown casual shoes or a comfy pair of athletic shoes. After you've satisfied the basic needs, start filling in as needed. But don't get too carried away. If your foot is still growing, you may outgrow shoes before you wear them!

Size

Have both feet sized by a professional:

    Right Foot Size:
    Left Foot Size:

Special Needs

Do your feet have any special needs? If you have your shoes professionally sized and still have trouble getting a comfortable fit, you might want to see if your feet are plagued with any of these potential problems.

Narrow Feet: People with narrow feet have a difficult time wearing regular width shoes; they feel big and cumbersome.

Wide Feet: Wide-footed people have a difficulty fitting into regular width shoes; their feet feel tight and restricted.

Flat Feet: People with flat feet experience pain in the arches of their feet due to lack of curvature.

Corns: Hard and soft (pea-sized) corns are found on or between toes and will cause great discomfort when pressure is applied.

Athlete's Foot: This fungus causes itching, redness, blisters, and cracking of skin.

Ingrown Toenail: Ingrown toenails cause pain due to cutting the toenails too round or too low. Toenails should be cut straight across, never at a curve.

Plantar Wart: This is a yellowish wart that grows on the sole of the foot and makes walking painful.

Bunion: Bunions are large protruding bumps on the inner border of the big toe joints. They incline the large toe towards the small one and are almost always caused by wearing poor-fitting shoes.

Watch Your Step

How do you put your foot down when you walk or run? Do you land on the ball of your foot or the heel of your foot? Do you place the majority of your weight on the outside or inside of your foot? Understanding the way you walk or run will enable you to purchase shoes with these needs in mind.

What to Buy

Write down the type and color of shoes you are interested in.

    Start with the basics and then expand from there:
    Kind:
    Color:
    Kind:
    Color:
    Kind:
    Color:

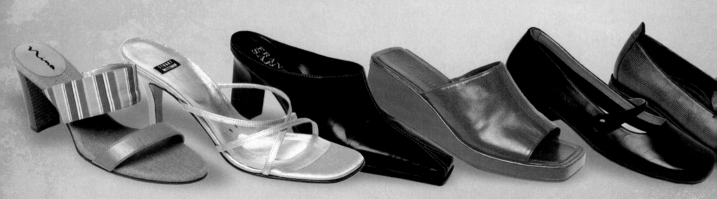

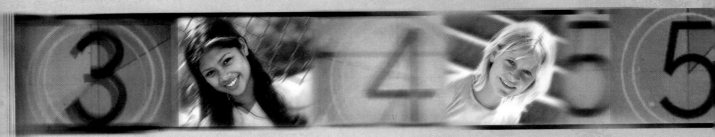

Part Two—
Peace for All Occasions

There are shoes made for all occasions, opportunities, and obstacles. Ballerinas wear slippers, baseball players wear spikes, and businesswomen wear pumps. You can even buy needle-spiked mountain climbing shoes to scale icy peaks! Different shoes can help you accomplish diverse tasks. With the right footwear, you can get a foothold on the objective at hand. ✳ Did you know that proper footwear is so important that God refers to it in the Bible? Following his Word, I'm going to show you how you can have beautiful feet without spending a fortune on foot spas, pedicures, or fancy footwear. Sit back, get comfy, and read the good news!

One of my favorite Bible verses talks about beautiful feet.

Isaiah 52:7—How beautiful on the mountains are the feet of those who bring good news, who proclaim peace, who bring good tidings, who proclaim salvation. . . .

I don't know about you, but I think of beautiful feet as pampered, polished, and buffed, resting comfortably on a stack of fluffy pillows. Yet those aren't the feet described in this passage. These feet are tired, sweaty, and

"Beautiful are the feet that bring good news!"

exhausted, persevering for the sake of delivering the good news about Jesus. Beautiful feet belong to those who share their relationship with Jesus Christ. I know this sounds a little intimidating, but I'm going to help you overcome these anxiety attacks in just two easy steps.

You'll be thrilled to know that God, the master designer, has fashioned a pair of shoes as part of your armor.

Ephesians 6:15— . . . and with your feet fitted with the readiness that comes from the gospel of peace.

I like to call these shoes "peace pumps" or "good news shoes"—the all-occasion footwear manufactured to peacefully scale obstacles and seize opportunities.

Soulful Solutions

Romans 5:1 (NKJV)—Therefore, having been justified by faith, we have peace with God through our Lord Jesus Christ.

Once you've accepted Jesus into your life, you immediately receive God's peace. It's not the kind of peace the world talks about; it's a reconciliation between you and the Prince of Peace himself—Jesus. The moment you begin a personal relationship with Jesus, you're given the armor of God, including the shoes of peace. They are the perfect fit, so let's try them on for size.

> **Display God's present of peace in your life by presenting the gospel through the way you live.**

Step #1—Size It Up

Romans 10:15 (NKJV)—"How beautiful are the feet of those who preach the gospel of peace, Who bring glad tidings of good things!"

As a Christian, the peace of God abides in you. The question is, do you live it? Others are constantly watching to see how your relationship with Jesus affects the way you behave.

Romans 10:15 states, "How beautiful are the feet of those who *preach* the gospel of peace." The word *preach* sounds a little scary, but what about the word *presents?* You'll make a great impression when you present the Lord to others just by living for him. Actions really do speak louder than words. Living life according to God's plan will give you the opportunity to share the gospel of peace!

Philippians 4:7 (CEV)—Then, because you belong to Christ Jesus, God will bless you with peace that no one can completely understand. And this peace will control the way you think and feel.

Step #2—Try It On for Size

The way you respond to your circumstances is a testimony to your faith in Christ. You can have a great witness by the way you react to difficult problems, by displaying peace during the ups and downs of life.

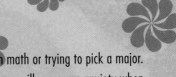

Can you think of a situation where a little peace would come in handy? Maybe you're struggling in math or trying to pick a major. Maybe you're at odds with your parents, or they're on the brink of divorce. Whatever the case, God's peace will overcome anxiety when you put your trust in him. But wearing your peace pumps is a choice. You can either choose to have God's peace in your life by drawing on his strength through prayer and Bible knowledge, or you can go it alone and hope for the best. I recommend you do it God's way.

Romans 15:13—May the God of hope fill you with all joy and peace as you trust in him, so that you may overflow with hope by the power of the Holy Spirit.

Scripture It

Leading by example is the most effective way to bring others to Christ. When you act out your faith, others will get a firsthand look at what a relationship with Jesus means. They'll see someone who makes mistakes but finds reconciliation, who faces temptation but draws strength from the Holy Spirit to overcome, and who faces turmoil but perseveres. Your example may be the only chance for someone to see what it means to have God's peace.

1 Timothy 4:12 (CEV)—Don't let anyone make fun of you, just because you are young. Set an example for other followers by what you say and do, as well as by your love, faith, and purity.

Although the apostle Paul wrote this verse to his young friend Timothy many years ago, I want to pass it along to you today. You are special, and don't let anyone tell you otherwise. I'm tired of society giving you no credit. The general public esteems you as irresponsible and addresses you like you can't be taught any better. When something goes wrong, many people say, "Well, what did we expect, after all they are only teenagers." How degrading!

I think we usually get what we expect. So if people expect more from teens, they'll receive more. And I believe you can do more than society gives you credit for! According to 1 Timothy 4:12, God expects you to be your best so you can be an example in all you say and do.

I know that the things you face are a lot more difficult than what I faced as a teen, but I also know that with God, you can handle the most challenging of circumstances. He equips us to endure life's hardest problems and promises us that he will never give us more than he enables us to handle.

1 Corinthians 10:13 (MESSAGE)—No test or temptation that comes your way is beyond the course of what others have had to face. All you need to remember is that God will never let you down; he'll never let you be pushed past your limit; he'll always be there to help you come through it.

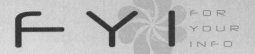

Let's talk about some ways you can share your relationship with Jesus by showing love and acceptance to others. It doesn't take much to be above average when it comes to being nice. Below is a list of ideas you can use to show kindness to others.

Send or give a card for no special reason.

Write a thank-you note to a teacher for helping you learn.

Pray for someone who offends you.

Bake some cookies for a friend.

Say thank you to the lunch staff at school.

Be friendly and courteous to the salesclerk at the mall.

Offer to let someone cut in front of you in line.

Compliment someone on what they are wearing.

Be nice to the new kid at school.

Smile and express thanks to the school bus driver for getting you to and from school safely.

Help out at home without being asked.

These seemingly small acts of kindness will set you apart from others. People will notice that there's something different about you, and this can present opportunities to share your faith in God. I'm not talking about preaching a sermon. I'm talking about simply acknowledging the source. For example, let's say you are nice to the kid at school who typically goes unnoticed. After a while, that person is going to wonder why you're nice and may even ask you about it. Here's your chance. You say, "I just think it's the right thing to do. Hey, by the way, you want to go to a youth thing at my church sometime?" How easy is that? Had you ever thought about sharing your faith just by being nice?

Super Models fashion their feet in peace.

✳ What This Means 2U

Securing your feet in God's famous footwear will keep you ready to share the Good News. The task will no longer seem undoable because God's supportive footgear motivates you to display the peace you have through your relationship with Jesus. When you mentally prepare yourself, you can move forward in your testimony instead of running away from the responsibility.

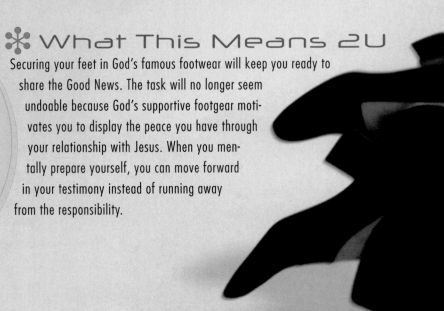

If you were off to play in a soccer tournament you would put on soccer shoes, wouldn't you? Well, guess what? Every day you play the most important game there is: the game of life. To be prepared, you need to study God's Word and pray. And you need to dress yourself in the armor of God so you are mentally, emotionally, and physically ready to play your best. So put on your peace pumps and get ready to go!

Test It Out

When you try on God's peace by accepting his salvation, you'll find out how well it fits and benefits every area of your life. God's peace not only reconciles you with him, it will also calm your fears and anxieties and help you face everyday adventures with an optimistic outlook. Let the peace of God rule in your heart, soul, and mind.

Pray and ask God for peace in all circumstances.

Examine what the Bible says about peace.

Act out your testimony by being kind.

Choose to apply God's peace in all you say and do.

Explore effective ways you can share the Good News.

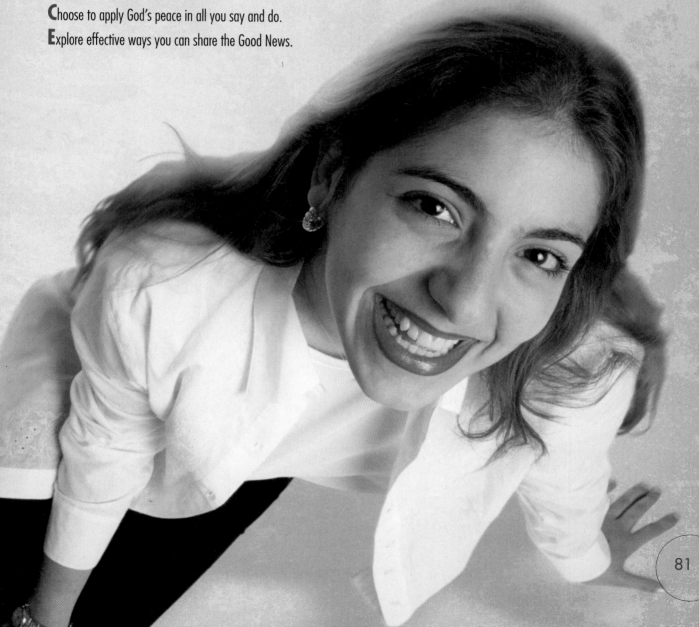

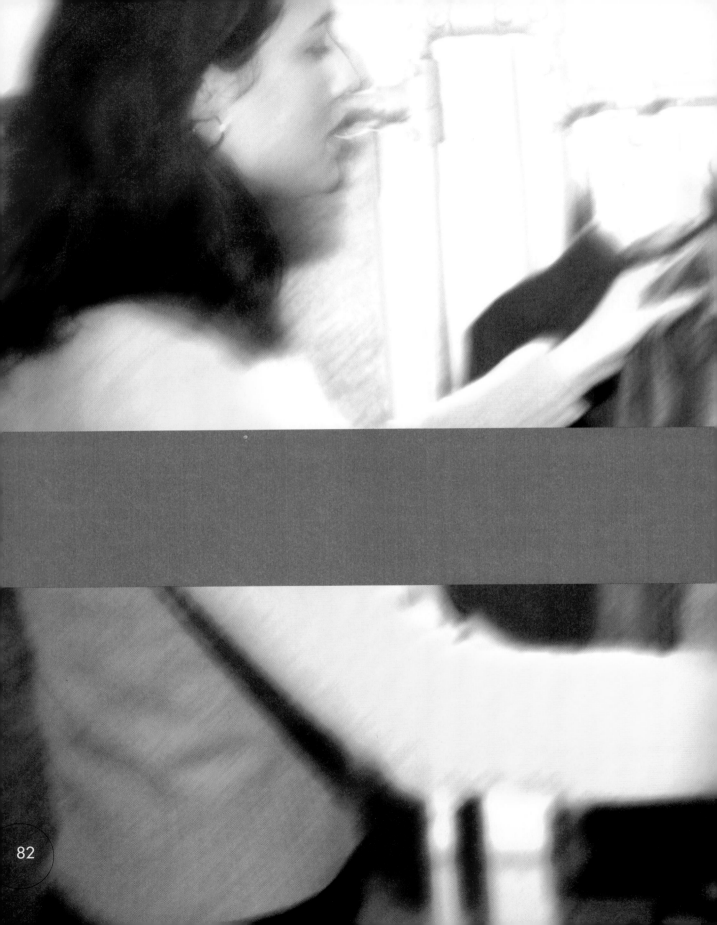

Style Savvy

Part One—Fashion Frenzy

Fashion is everywhere. No matter where you turn you're bombarded with the latest and greatest designs. We see it at the mall, in magazines, on television, at school, even at church. Our trendsetting environment impacts how we view fashion and how we dress. We just can't escape outside influences. So how can we still dress with individuality without going broke? ✳ In this chapter, we'll learn how to shield ourselves from uniformity by applying a touch of personal style to our clothing. We'll shield ourselves from overspending by learning how to shop sensibly and mix and match wardrobe separates. And finally, we'll discover what it means to shield ourselves with compassion. ✳ Are you ready to replace fashion faux pas with fashion freedom? Then keep reading.

Do you have to dress trendy in order to be a trendsetter? Absolutely not. In fact, dressing trendy is just falling prey to the ideas of high-profile designers. I often wonder if these people sit around a large conference table and take a vote on how they'll torment women over the course of another year. I imagine one designer saying, "I vote for narrow-toed shoes that will make their feet hurt," and another saying, "I vote for tight jeans that will cut off their circulation when they sit down." After they talk, they put it to vote, and the latest trends are born.

Maybe it doesn't exactly work this way, but I know one thing for sure: We've been programmed to buy whatever the fashion experts say we should. As soon as trends hit the stores we race off to pay top dollar for something we don't really want in the first place. So why do we fall for it? It's because we have an innate need to fit in. This isn't necessarily a bad thing, but it can have adverse affects if we aren't careful.

So, how can we cover ourselves without suffering the consequences of poor design? The solution is in the shield.

✳ Simple Solutions

Step #1—Shield Yourself from Uniformity

Shield yourself from uniformity by applying personal style to your wardrobe.

What is your *personal style?* What sets you apart from others in the way you dress or express yourself? Maybe you've never thought about this before, but I'm going to help you figure out the answers.

So what does it take to be you? Only you can answer that question. Maybe it means being associated with a group of some sort—a sports team, a school, a hobby. I knew a girl who loved the Washington Redskins. It didn't matter what she wore, it had something to do with the team insignia or colors. My daughter, who surfs for a hobby, frequently wears clothing that shows a surfing logo. Both of these girls show *personal style* in the way they dress. Personally, I love glamour and glitz! Give me anything that makes my wardrobe shine and I'm happy!

Let's say your teacher walks in one day and says, "The school is putting a dress code into effect and everyone will wear uniforms." The only difference between you and everyone else will lie in your own *personal style (P.S.).* Your *P.S.* will interpret how you decide to wear the uniform. Will you have fun with it and glitz it up a bit? Or will you make it work by adding a necktie? Maybe you'll starch it, iron it, and perfect it with just the right belt and matching loafers. Whatever the look, the choice is yours; it's all about *personal style.*

Personal style is the difference between **trendy** and trendsetter.

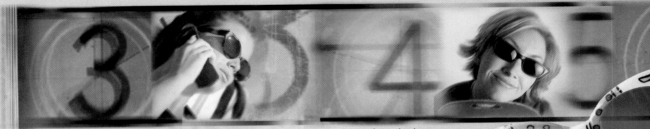

Your *P.S.* will change as interests vary and time evolves, but don't let that stop you from displaying who you are right now. Take comfort in who you are and others will be comfortable with you too.

What is your *P.S.* (personal style)? What would you like it to be?

_____

How will you develop it?

_____

Step #2—Shield Yourself from Overspending

Shield yourself from overspending by learning how to mix and match your wardrobe.

Knowing how to mix and match wardrobe separates will save you time and allow variety without stuffing your dresser drawers or going broke. Start with the basics and then add extras. You don't have to own a lot of clothes to have a large wardrobe. When you wear colors from your color family your clothing will naturally blend, making mixing and matching easy.

I'd begin with the basics: two or three pairs of jeans (one trendy pair and a pair or two that are not too trendy), a pair of khakis, and one other pair of neutral-colored pants such as gray, navy, or black. Then I'd add a denim or khaki skirt and a sundress that could be easily accessorized for winter wear. Next, add three or four interchangeable tops, a couple of cardigans, and a jacket or blazer. These will start your new school year with a minimum of thirty-nine outfits to mix and match. That means you can go a whole month and never wear the same combination twice!

You may be wondering if thirteen to fourteen garments can really put together a decent wardrobe. The answer is yes—especially when you start adding accessories. I don't know about you, but I get into clothing ruts where I wear the same outfits over and over again because I know they look good and I don't have to put much thought into getting dressed. Even if your closet and dresser drawers are jam-packed with clothes, you'll probably find that you wear what's easily accessible. It's easier than trying to come up with something new to wear on the spur of the moment.

My P.S. includes wearing different colored **sunglasses** that match my outfits.

85

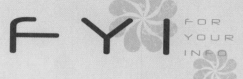

Step #3—Shield Yourself from Paying Retail

Shield yourself from paying retail by learning how to be a savvy shopper.

Shopping can be rewarding and fun if you do it right. I am an infamous bargain shopper. I don't believe in paying full price for anything. I love browsing the malls, but I rarely find any real deals unless there are clearance sales going on. But I'd rather buy my summer fashions in the summer season rather than the fall. So I usually shop at discount stores like T.J. Maxx, Marshalls, Stein Mart, the Nordstrom Rack (Nordstrom Outlet), or thrift shops.

I like to call this scavenger shopping because you never know what you might find. The trick is making these stores work to your advantage. Let's say you see a really great got-to-have-it outfit at the mall or in the catalog. First, either tear the page from the catalog or make a mental note of what the outfit at the mall looked like. Then head off to a discount store or thrift shop to put together the same type of outfit.

I once found a sensational outfit in a catalog for $309. I took the picture and was able to find a similar outfit for only $39.97 at T.J. Maxx. And when I went to a thrift shop, I was able to put together the same outfit for just $13.50, a savings of $295.50!

Step #4—Shield Yourself with Loving-Kindness

Shield yourself with loving-kindness; the same type of compassion you would like to be shown.

"Do unto others as you would have them do unto you." This is known as the Golden Rule; it doesn't ask any more or any less of you than what you want to receive. If you are willing to accept intolerance, hate, and criticism then dish it out. But if you want others to treat you with respect and hold you in high regard, then do the same to them. There's an old saying, "What goes around, comes around," and I've found this to be very true. You can't plant carrot seeds and receive green beans, just as you can't plant contempt and expect compassion in return.

Beauty pageants often select Miss Congeniality, someone who represents the heart of inner beauty. This person is well-liked due to her genuine compassion towards the other contestants. She doesn't allow the contest to stand in the way of esteeming others. To me, this award speaks higher of a woman's beauty than the actual Miss "Whoever" crown does.

Strive to model congeniality and I'll guarantee you this; you'll be valued far above the winner of any beauty pageant. When you touch the hearts and lives of others, you reward yourself in return.

✳ **What This Means 2U** Keeping yourself dressed in the latest fashions can make your head spin if you don't apply a little common sense when you go shopping. Wearing the right clothes, especially what's right for you, is important to your self-confidence. We all like to dress right, look right, and feel right in our outward appearance, but never allow that to overshadow who you are on the inside. Contrary to popular belief, clothes do not

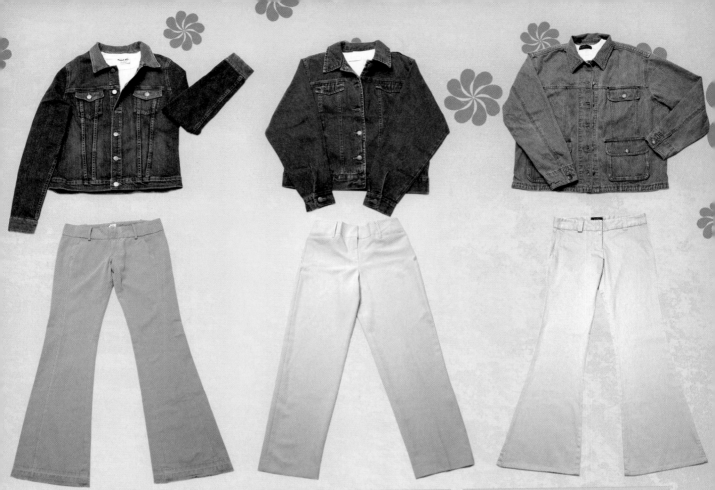

#1 Original Designer Outfit
Purchased at Nordstrom

- Hudson Denim Jacket $143.00
- Joie Khakis   130.00
- Michael Stars Tee   36.00

Total $309.00

#2 Designer Knock-Off
Purchased at T.J. Maxx

- Bill Blass Denim Jacket $12.99
- Larry Levine Khakis   16.99
- Lizwear Tee   9.99

Total $39.97

SAVINGS OF   **$269.03**

#3 Thrift Shop Knock-Off
Purchased at The Second Hand

- St. John Bay Denim Jacket $6.00
- Zinc Khakis (new with tags!)   4.50
- Karen Scott Tee   3.00

Total $13.50

SAVINGS OF   **$295.50**

make the person; friendliness does. Don't make fun of anyone for the way they dress. And avoid stereotyping people because of out-of-date clothing or poor personal hygiene. It's who we are on the inside that really counts.

❧Test It Out

You've learned a lot in this chapter, and now it's time to put it to use. It's one thing to know it, but it's another thing to apply it. First, take time to develop your own personal style. Second, learn to mix and match separates to create a seemingly endless wardrobe. Third, be a smart shopper. And finally, treat others the way you want to be treated. Put these ideas into practice, and you'll shield yourself from fashion fallout.

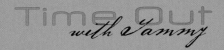

Time Out
with Tammy

I learned at an early age what it means to view a person for who they are on the inside instead of what they wear on the outside. In first grade, I met Dianna, a skinny, freckle-faced girl with long, tangled hair. Everyone, including me, made fun of Dianna because she wore old, ratty clothes that were either too big or too small for her frail frame.

One day while I was with my great-aunt making invitations for my birthday party, I told her to write one for everyone in my class except Dianna. Auntie asked me why, and I told her. "She's poor, and she wears ugly clothes that look like rags. Nobody likes her." Auntie got tears in her eyes and said, "Tammy Susan, I don't ever want to hear you talk like that again. That little girl can't help the way she dresses, and do you know how I know that? I was once that little girl. I grew up in a very poor family and only had two dresses to my name. My shoes had holes in the soles and the only underwear I had were so stretched out that I had to keep them up with pins. All the teasing hurt so much that I quit school after the sixth grade. I'm sure Dianna doesn't like the way she dresses either, but if her parents can't afford pretty clothes for her to wear that doesn't make her a bad person. I want you to remember that and be extra nice to her from now on."

The next day I went to school clothed with a new attitude. I asked Dianna to be my friend. I remember vividly the first time she came over to my house to play. We were playing Barbie's when she told me that she didn't want to kill herself anymore because she had a friend. Before then, I had never known anyone who wanted to kill themselves before, and yet here was Dianna sitting right next to me and telling me how she went home from school every day wishing to die. She told me that she even took a butcher knife from the drawer one day and contemplated stabbing herself. And why? Just because kids made fun of her for the way she dressed.

Girls of all ages are affected by mean words; they hurt feelings and destroy lives. How do your words affect others?

As you learn how to develop your own personal style by mixing and matching your wardrobe at a savings, keep in mind the most important shield of all; the shield of compassion.

> I love the thrill of the hunt when I go thrift store shopping. Once I found a $3750 **designer fur** (the original price tag was still in the pocket) in a clearance bin at a resale shop for only $25!

No Uniformity

Shield yourself from uniformity by applying personal style to your wardrobe.

Answer the questions below to help determine your personal style.

Are you a fan of any particular sports team?   Y   N   Team:

Are you a fan of any particular school?   Y   N   School:

What are your hobbies or interests?

Which method of dress do you prefer?

> Colorful, glittery fashion
>
> Task-oriented clothing
>
> Perfectly-pressed shirt and pants
>
> Comfort first

If there is one thing you could add to your wardrobe, what would it be?

Use the answers above to determine your personal style.

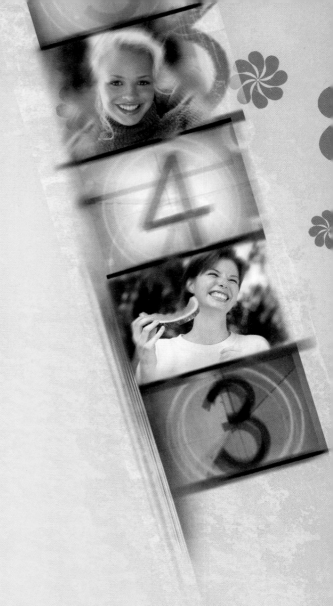

No Overspending

Avoid overspending by learning how to mix and match your wardrobe.

Do you have the basics?

> 1 pair of trendy jeans
>
> 2 pairs of (not too trendy) jeans
>
> 1 pair of khakis
>
> 1 pair of neutral pants (gray, navy, or black)
>
> 1 denim or khaki skirt
>
> 1 sundress
>
> 3–4 interchangeable tops
>
> 2 cardigans
>
> 1 jacket or blazer

No Paying Retail

Learn how to be a savvy shopper. Do your own comparison-shopping. The next time you see that can't-live-without-it outfit in the mall or in a magazine, put scavenger shopping to the test.

Nothing But Loving-Kindness

Regard others the way you would like to be regarded.

Is there anyone you need to be nicer to?

How will you make an effort to esteem this person?

Record the results here:

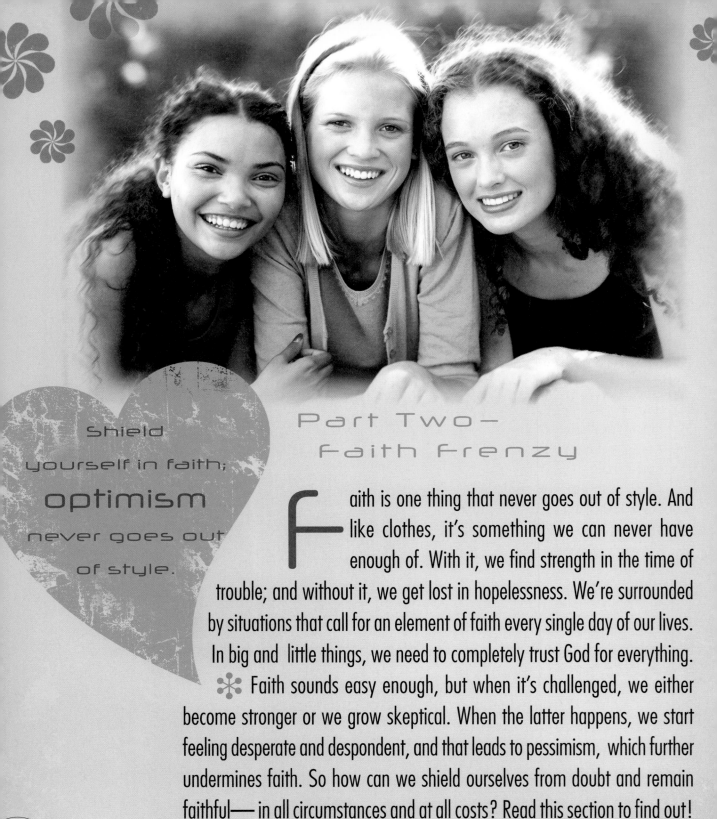

Part Two—
Faith Frenzy

Shield yourself in faith; **optimism** never goes out of style.

Faith is one thing that never goes out of style. And like clothes, it's something we can never have enough of. With it, we find strength in the time of trouble; and without it, we get lost in hopelessness. We're surrounded by situations that call for an element of faith every single day of our lives. In big and little things, we need to completely trust God for everything.

❋ Faith sounds easy enough, but when it's challenged, we either become stronger or we grow skeptical. When the latter happens, we start feeling desperate and despondent, and that leads to pessimism, which further undermines faith. So how can we shield ourselves from doubt and remain faithful—in all circumstances and at all costs? Read this section to find out!

You must practice faith in order to remain faithful. Of course, faith is easier to talk about than to live out. It's like exercise; talking about it won't do a bit of good, but when it's practiced, we reap the benefits. It gives us the strength we need to carry on.

God's got you covered even when you're unaware of his presence. He's faithful 24/7; the question is how can we exercise *our* faith in him? Just like exercise, we must take it up to make it work; so *take up* the shield of faith.

Ephesians 6:16—In addition to all this, take up the shield of faith, with which you can extinguish all the flaming arrows of the evil one.

Soulful Solutions

Step #1—Shield Yourself from Underestimation

Shield yourself from underestimating the power you have through the Holy Spirit living in you.

2 Timothy 1:7 (CEV)—God's Spirit doesn't make cowards out of us. The Spirit gives us power, love, and self-control.

Do you remember the cowardly lion in the Wizard of Oz? The lion, king of the jungle, asked the wizard to grant him courage, confidence, and self-control. The wizard, a man of wisdom, helped the lion find the power deep within himself; he found confidence and faith he didn't even know he possessed.

How many times have you felt like the lion—like you possess the power, but lack the confidence or self-control to shield yourself with it? We underestimate the influence of the Holy Spirit living within us. He can help us and empower us through faith. Through prayer, we can gain courage to face life. Through trials, we gain confidence in who we are in Jesus Christ. And through time, the Holy Spirit helps us gain self-control. As Christians, our faith shields us from underestimating the Holy Spirit's power to give us courage, confidence, and self-control.

Scripture It

Step #2—Shield Yourself from the Opposition

Shield yourself from the opposition by using common sense.

Proverbs 3:21–22 (CEV)—My child, use common sense and sound judgment! Always keep them in mind. They will help you to live a long and beautiful life.

In biblical times, Roman soldiers carried shields made of wood and iron that covered the height and width of their bodies. Soaked in water, the shields extinguished flaming arrows upon impact. Although the soldiers wore protective body armor, they mainly used the shields to put out fire. Most importantly, they had to keep the shield between them and the enemy to protect themselves.

Your shield of faith works the same way. It's designed to extinguish the fiery darts Satan tempts you with. Faith in God helps us look past the circumstances and weigh the consequences using good old common sense. But you must keep the shield between you and the enemy for it to be effective; never lay it aside or you'll become vulnerable and victimized.

There's an old saying, "If you can't stand the heat, stay out of the kitchen." These are good words when it comes to avoiding Satan's fiery arrows. If you can't handle a situation

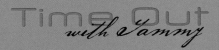

Time Out
with Tammy

While teaching a workshop, I met a gal named Rachel. After the session she asked if she could talk to me so we found a vacant area and sat down to chat. Rachel's eyes filled with tears and she started the conversation with, "If only I'd used my common sense and listened to my parents."

She and her boyfriend, Randy, had been an item for more than four months. Rachel wasn't allowed to date, but Randy was allowed to visit Rachel at her house as long as one of her parents was home. A few days after Randy got his driver's license he drove to school for the very first time. After school he asked Rachel if he could drive her home. She accepted the invitation and off they went. Once they got to Rachel's house, Randy asked to come in, but Rachel told him she wasn't allowed to have guests when her parents weren't home. Randy pushed the issue with, "Who's going to know? I'll leave before anyone comes home." The pit of Rachel's stomach grumbled "No," but Rachel went against her better judgment and said, "Okay."

Once inside, one thing led to another, and they started making out. But it didn't stop there. They went all the way. Afterwards, Rachel felt like an emotional wreck, sorry and confused. She hadn't planned on or wanted to have sex. But one thing led to another and it happened. The next day at school, Randy treated the situation like it was no big deal. Instead of feeling loved, Rachel felt used and ashamed. About a week later Rachel and Randy broke up. But, unfortunately that's not the end of the story. Those few moments of quick sex left Rachel burdened with guilt, bouts of depression, and the Herpes Simplex Virus—a painful and incurable STD.

Rachel's plea for help wasn't what you might think. Though she still suffered from the physical consequences of sin, she has found peace by praying and asking God for forgiveness. She asked me to pass her story on in hope that others won't become "if only" victims, living in regret. So keep your faith strong through prayer and Bible study, and use your common sense to live a long and beautiful life.

or you're not prepared to deal with the consequences, don't even go there. Don't put yourself into a tempting situation by laying your shield down and walking into the enemy camp.

Have you ever chosen to put yourself into a circumstance, even though your gut warned you against it? We're all guilty of this at some time. I don't know how many times I've heard, "If only I'd gone with my gut feeling," or "If only I'd used common sense." Unfortunately, we never say this until it's too late.

There are two kinds of "if onlies" in life; the kind you can control, and the kind you can't. Using common sense, you can control lots of "if onlies." For example, good sense tells you to study for a test so that you won't fail and say, "If only I'd studied for the test . . ." But some "if onlies" are more about wishful thinking than common sense; "If only I could win a million dollars." Wishful thinking tells us there are no consequences to our actions and we can find the easy way out. Unfortunately, I think we often apply wishful thinking instead of common sense.

Step #3—Shield Yourself from Praying Reluctantly

Shield yourself from praying reluctantly by remembering answered prayers.

James 1:6–7 (CEV)—But when you ask for something, you must have faith and not doubt. Anyone who doubts is like an ocean wave tossed around in a storm. If you are that kind of person, you can't make up your mind, and you surely can't be trusted. So don't expect the Lord to give you anything at all.

Faith is key to answered prayer. When we pray expectantly we can be sure of an answer. But according to James 1:6–7, when we pray with wishy-washy faith we can't expect to receive anything from the Lord. I do believe it's possible to pray in bewilderment, not knowing how to specifically pray for something. But as long as you pray in faith, knowing there will be an answer of some sort, then you are still praying in confidence of God. Faith means we should completely trust God for the answer, whether we like it or not.

Sometimes, though, it's difficult to have faith. Some situations seem overwhelming and hopeless. But answered prayer is a faith-building experience. When you feel your faith fading, sit down and think about the prayers God has answered in the past. As you remember the cool things he's done before, you'll find your faith growing and remain confident that he can answer future prayers.

When God **answers** my prayer, I date it, record the outcome, and highlight it for future reference.

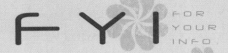

FYI
FOR YOUR INFO.

I don't know about you, but I can be extremely absentminded when it comes to remembering answered prayer. I'm overjoyed when it happens, and I'm quick to thank God, but let a few days pass and I'm back to my bout with doubt where other prayer requests are concerned. It was easy to forget about God's answers to prayer, until I started writing them down. I began journaling my prayer requests and recording the answers.

Whenever I start to question whether or not God is still in the prayer-answering business, I open my prayer diary and read over the prayers he's already answered. When I stop and reflect, I'm always amazed at God's faithfulness to me. At the same time, my faith in God grows, enabling my shield of faith to douse the darts of doubt Satan fires at me.

✳ What This Means 2U
Never underestimate the power of the Spirit to lead you into bold faith. Use common sense and keep the shield positioned between you and the enemy. Don't lay it aside, even for a moment, or the enemy is sure to attack. But if you do get off course, pray and ask God to forgive your faithlessness and to help you make wiser decisions in the future. Exercising good prayer practices by journaling your requests and answers will also help you remain faithful to God.

But remember, even after you do all these things, you need to activate your faith shield.

James 2:17—Faith by itself, if it is not accompanied by action, is dead.

Don't be a deadbeat; exercise faith. Your faith is a living, breathing testament of what it means to have a relationship with Christ. Even though our actions don't earn us a spot in heaven, they do convey that our devotion to God is real. Exercising faith by serving God may be the very example someone needs to witness in order to believe.

Unquestionably, living our faith is one of the toughest things we're called to do. Living by faith goes against our human nature, even when we know Christ personally. It's all about trust. And the Spirit will help you exercise it, practice it, and live by it.

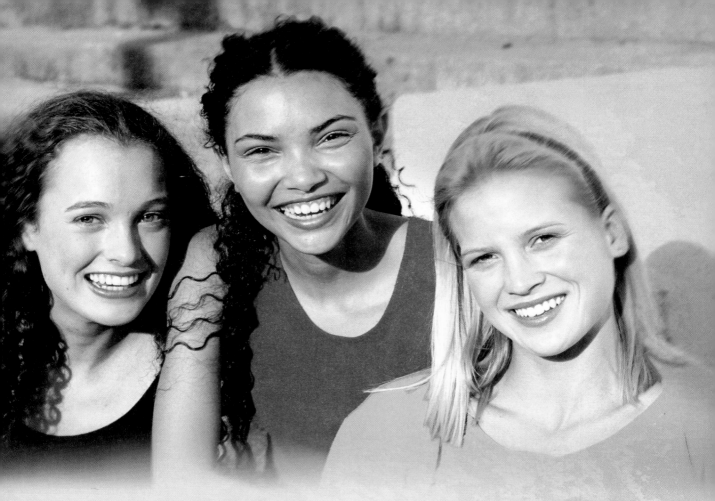

❧Test It Out

Faith is something you can easily put to the test. First, exercise the power you have through the Holy Spirit. He'll help you find courage, confidence, and self-control in Christ. Second, keep yourself covered in faith, using common sense to protect you from the devil's faith-shattering darts. Third, pray in faith, expecting an answer. You serve a big God, so the greater the request, the grander the response. And finally, don't sit on these suggestions—activate them!

Fully rely on God.

Always pray expecting an answer.

Initiate the power of the Holy Spirit living in you.

Track your prayer progress in a journal.

Honor God by using common sense and sound judgment.

Super Models **shield** themselves in faith.

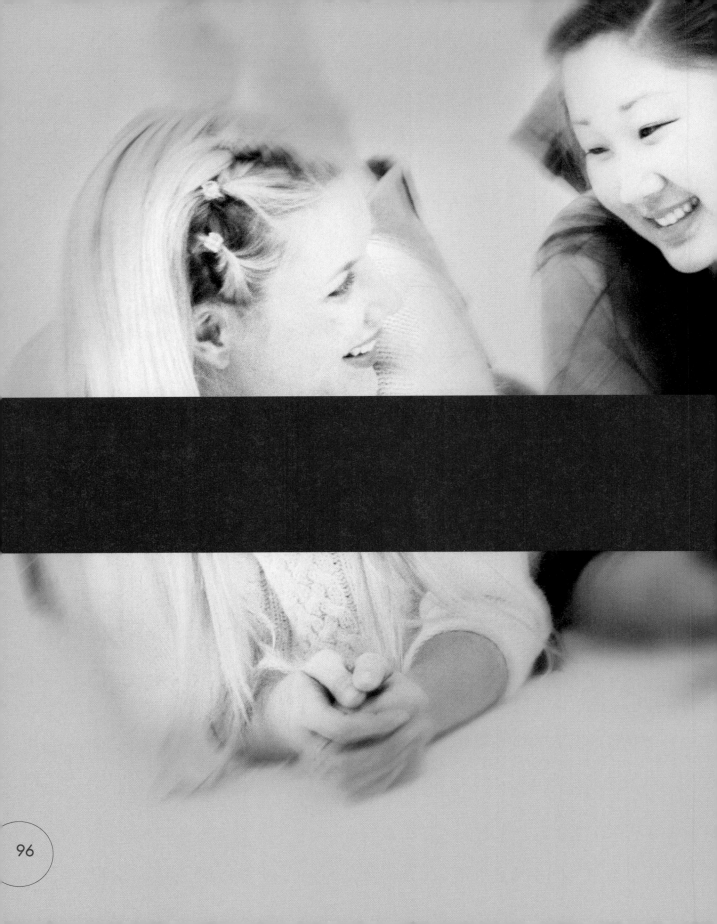

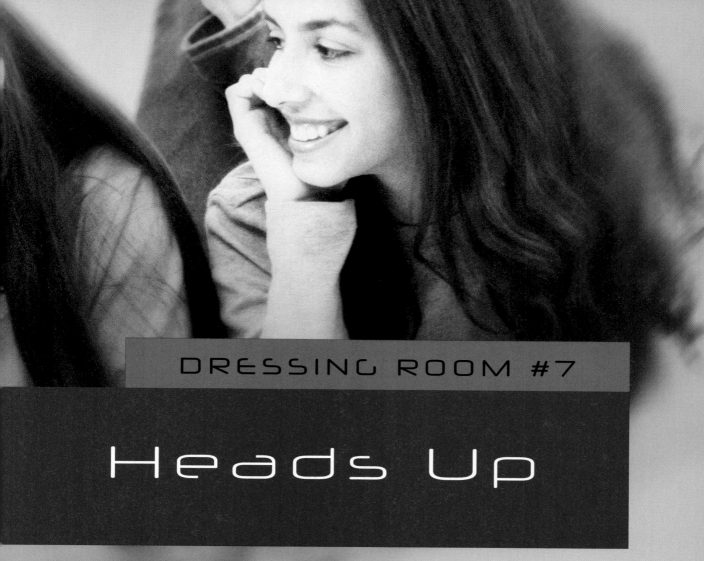

Heads Up

Part One—Hats Off

I t's time to get the heads up on fashion. Our clothes are significant, but we can't pull off a complete look without focusing on how we dress from the neck up. Your face is the focal point of communication, and others notice what they see there. ❋ But your real value isn't in your wardrobe; it comes out through your conversation and carriage. It's important to project a positive attitude, allowing everything on the outside to accessorize the real beauty on the inside. And since inner beauty is conveyed most often from the neck up, it's essential that your face and hair look their very best.

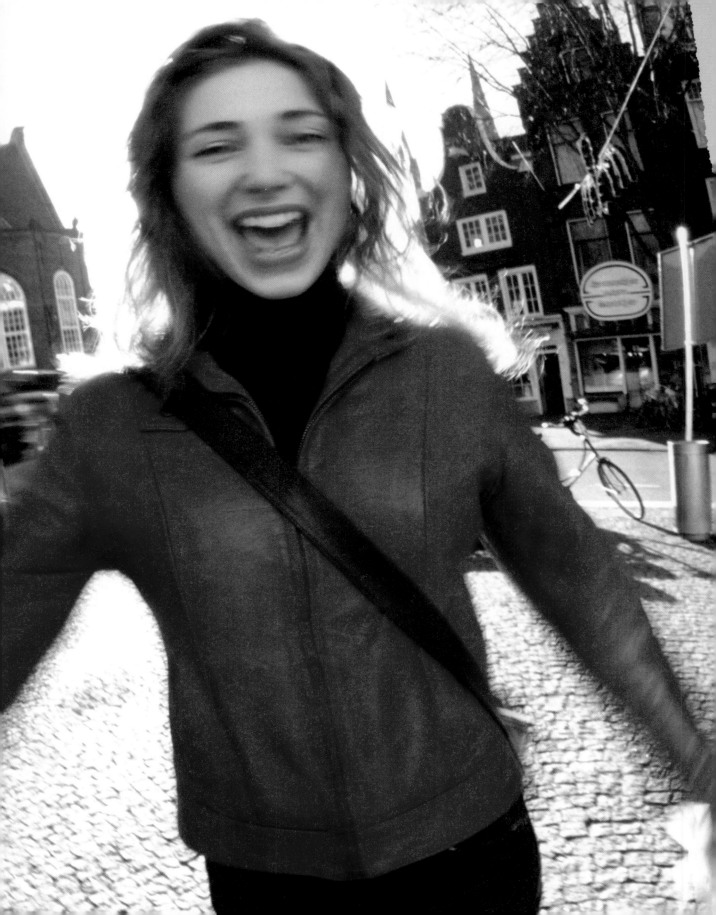

How many of you have experienced the following scenario? You're lounging around the house, sweats on, hair uncombed, no makeup on, when your mom invites you to go to the store with her. You hesitate for a second because of your sloppy appearance and then you think, "Well, I need to pick up some deodorant, and who's going to see me anyway?" Then, when you arrive at the store, you seem to run into everyone you know!

Sneaking out of the house looking less-than-decent is like sending out an invitation to meet everyone we know wherever we're going. And to add insult to injury, we usually run into that one person we especially don't want to see us when we're at our worst!

I've learned from experience to at least have my hair combed and minimal makeup on when I go out. What I'm wearing isn't as important to my self-assurance as my point of communication— my face and, of course, great attitude and winning smile makes a winning combination with anyone you run into.

❋ Simple Solutions

We all want great-looking faces, thus the reason for multibillion dollar beauty industries. But how can we cater to our desires and avoid the confusion and the cost?

Two simple steps will achieve a great-looking face.

Flatter It

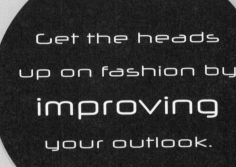

Develop a skin care program that flatters your skin type.

A simple skin care routine, based on the needs of your skin type (dry, normal, oily, combination, or sensitive) will refresh your skin and give it a healthy glow. Start and end your day with a cleanser that deep cleans and freshens your skin, followed by a toner to remove excess dirt and restore the pH balance. Finish with a moisturizer to replenish and protect your skin. Once a week, use an exfoliant to slough off the dead skin cells that clog your pores and cause breakouts.

The right cleanser, toner, moisturizer, and exfoliant will improve any skin type. If you need information to determine the needs of your skin, read the first chapter of my book about beauty. You'll find everything you need to know about establishing a skin care routine that is right for you.

Finish It

Finish your face with cosmetics that complement your skin tone.

Once you've cared for your skin properly, you're ready for cosmetics. Makeup enhances your facial features and improves any wardrobe. Whether you're wearing a striking dress or scruffy jeans, healthy skin and pretty makeup complement what you wear.

When choosing makeup, start with the basics—a sheer foundation to even out your skin tone and an opaque concealer to cover imperfections on your skin. Follow up with a bit of blush, eye makeup, and a light dusting of translucent powder. Put on some lip gloss, and you're finished!

The great thing about makeup is that you can change your look to go along with any occasion or outfit. Are you going to a football game? Then wear eye shadows in your school colors and paint a football on your cheek. Or maybe you're going to homecoming. Intensify your makeup for the evening and add a splash of glitter on your cheeks, eyes, and shoulders.

Cosmetics are fun to experiment with, but never overdo it. Successful makeup is worn without looking all made up. If you'd like more information on applying makeup that's right for you, refer to my book about beauty.

Time Out
with Tammy

I have a heart-shaped face that is well pronounced by the widow's peak at the top of my forehead. For years, I hated my widow's peak and even used tweezers to pluck the hairs out because kids teased me. I felt like a freak of nature. Little did I know then that widow's peaks are often considered beauty marks.

People who dish out cruel comments have their own insecurities. They think that they have to make fun of other people in order to make themselves look good. Don't fall for it. Be comfortable with who you are, and others will be comfortable with you too, even if they initially tease you. Be a Super Model; be above average by modeling what it means to build someone up instead of tearing them down.

PICTURE IT 54

The choicest accessory to any wardrobe isn't something you need to search for, but something you already possess—your hair. Smart, sassy, short, or straight, your lovely locks hold the key to a successful look.

Frame It

Frame your face with a hairstyle that fits its shape.

Have you ever had your hair styled like someone else's only to discover that it didn't look nearly as good on you? Or did you ever use the same hair care products as the girl in the magazine without achieving the promised results? Finding a hairstyle that works with your face shape and hair texture requires some expertise and involves a little bit of artistic expression. But don't worry, I'm here to help.

The shape of your face determines whether you wear your hairstyle or your hairstyle wears you. Your hair should frame your facial features in a way that brings balance to the shape of your head. That's why your friend may look adorable in a wedge cut, while you look weird when you try it. Knowing your face helps to determine the right 'do for you.

Use the information provided below to match your shape with the best style.

Oval—Add volume around your cheekbones in order to create width and balance to your face's long shape. Hairstyles that feature layers or loose, tousled curls work best.

Rectangle—Add bangs to visually shorten your face's length and create width by adding volume around the cheekbones. Avoid styles that add height to the top of your head.

Square—Soften the edges with wispy rounded bangs or wavy layers that flatter your face. Avoid angular cuts or styles that add width to the jawline.

Round—Try long layered hairstyles or short-stacked haircuts that create height and elongate the face without adding width.

Heart—Minimize the width of the forehead with soft bangs or curls and add fullness at the jawline.

Fix It

Whether you want to fix the style or restore its shape, the right products will do wonders for your hair.

Finding the right hair care products is not only exasperating, it's also expensive. My vanity cabinet is full of partially used hair care products that I've used on a trial-and-error method. Use the following information to match your hair texture and feel to the right hair formula.

Dry—Dry hair is dull and brittle and tends to easily break off. It doesn't contain enough moisture due to weather, sun, chlorine, chemical processing, styling tools, or in some cases, medical conditions. You need a protein packet (found in most drugstores or beauty supply stores). Shampoo your hair with a moisturizing shampoo and then deep massage the entire protein packet into your hair. Put a plastic shower cap over your head and let it deep condition for at least thirty minutes. Don't worry about leaving it in too long; your hair will only absorb as much conditioner as it needs. When the time is up, rinse out the conditioner, towel dry, and then let your hair air dry the rest of the way. Never blow dry your hair; blow drying dries your hair out.

Rinsing your hair with cool water will help make it **shine**.

Oily—Whether it's because of menstrual, hormonal, or genetic factors, your scalp produces too much oil. Use a clarifying shampoo or a shampoo specially formulated for oily hair. When you wash your hair, concentrate on massaging the scalp because this is where the oil comes from.

Remember, always shampoo twice, once to break down the oil buildup, and a second time to wash it away. You may also want to avoid bangs because oily bangs can cause breakouts on your forehead.

Dull—If your hair is dull, flat, and lacks luster you're probably suffering from product overload or chlorine buildup. To restore your hair's shine use $1/4$ cup shampoo to 1 tablespoon baking soda. Mix together and then shampoo your hair twice. Use this formula once a week to maintain shiny hair.

Straight—Keep straight hair looking healthy by brushing it with a brush made of natural bristles such as boar's hair. Natural bristles are porous and spread the organic oils from your scalp throughout your hair to provide natural shine. To avoid frizz, spray your hair with a detangling product, use a large round brush, and blow dry your hair one section at a time.

Curly—Curly hair tends to dry out, frizz, and tangle easily. To combat those unruly locks, use a moisturizing shampoo and a leave-in conditioner. Comb through curly hair with a wide-toothed pick and let it air dry, or use a diffuser on your blow dryer to avoid frizz.

Fine—Use a volumizing shampoo and conditioner to give fine, limp hair a boost. For added body, apply mousse or root lifting gel at the base of your hair and then hold your head upside down and blow dry your hair. Still lacking body? Roll your hair with large Velcro rollers, spraying the roots with hairspray. Go over it with a hot blow dryer and then cool it off by giving it a shot with the cool button on your blow dryer. If you don't have a cool shot button, let it cool down naturally before you remove the rollers. Then remove the rollers and gently brush your hair into place with a vent hairbrush.

Coarse—Coarse hair tends to be thick, wiry, and hard to manage if you don't use the right products. Use a moisturizing shampoo and leave-in conditioner to keep your hair manageable, and apply a silicone-based frizz control serum to keep it smooth.

Hair Loss—Experiencing a certain amount of hair loss is perfectly normal. The average person loses 100–130 hairs a day. If you are experiencing severe hair loss, consult a physician. To promote hair growth, give yourself a three-minute scalp massage (using your fingertips, not your nails) when you shampoo your hair. This releases dead skin cells and stimulates blood flow to the hair follicles, encouraging new growth. A second method of scalp massage involves applying a leave-in conditioner to your hair and massaging it into your hair and scalp for five to ten minutes.

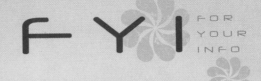

Fashion It

Refashion, redesign, and restyle yourself with a new haircut

One of the easiest and least expensive ways to get a new look is with a trendy new haircut. Whether you've been in a hair rut and need a change, or just want to get a trim, save yourself from haircut heartbreak by reading the information below.

Picture—A picture is worth a thousand words. Flip through magazines for hairstyle ideas, and when you find one, clip it and take it with you to the stylist. As you're searching for the right style, remember the texture of your hair and the shape of your face are the most important factors in choosing a manageable style.

Pick a Stylist—Picking a quality hair stylist can be difficult if you don't know what to look for. In the last twenty years I've moved a number of times, and every move has required me to choose a new hairdresser. Two rules of thumb that have helped me are: (1) If you see someone with great hair, ask her who she goes to, and (2) find a stylist that is Redken certified. Redken-certified stylists have to stay up to date on current trends, styles, and cuts in order to maintain their certification.

Person-to-Person—Ask for a consultation with the stylist before he or she begins. Having one-on-one time with the hairdresser can relieve nerves and give you an opportunity to ask questions while the stylist gets acquainted with your hair. Show the hairdresser the style you want and ask if it will work with your hair texture and face shape. Also find out if the style will require extra tools or products. If you're not comfortable with the stylist, don't go through with the service. Graciously tell the stylist you've changed your mind and find a hairdresser that you can trust. If you do get your hair done and are unhappy with it for any reason, be sure and let the hairdresser know. He or she should fix it to your satisfaction at no extra cost. If you're not sure about your new look because you've made a drastic change, wait a few days before asking to have it redone.

What This Means 2U

Although your hair, makeup, and skin care aren't considered wardrobe items, they are valuable assets to anything you wear. Fresh, healthy skin will set off every outfit. Remember, your wardrobe begins with your features and the attitude you model. Accentuate yourself from the top of your head to the tip of your toes to keep yourself looking good, and no matter what you wear, always try to display a positive attitude.

103

❯Test It Out

It's time to reevaluate what you've learned. Use the worksheet below to create a healthy skin care program and to pick cosmetics and hairstyles that are great on you. These are important aspects to looking your very best. And when you look good, you feel better about yourself and act more confident.

FLATTER IT

Develop a skin care program that flatters your skin type.

What type of skin do you have?

    DRY   NORMAL   OILY   COMBINATION

What type of cleanser do you use?

What type of toner do you use?

What type of moisturizer do you use?

What type of exfoliant do you use?

*Special Note: You should see positive results in the condition of your skin within ten days of using facial products.

FINISH IT

Finish your face with cosmetics that complement your skin tone.

Is your complexion

    LIGHT   MEDIUM   DARK

Which color family do you belong to?

    WARM   COOL

What type of skin do you have?

    DRY   NORMAL   OILY   COMBINATION

What is your skin texture?

    SOFT   SMOOTH   ROUGH   PITTED   SCARRED   ACNE-PRONE   OTHER

The answers to all of these questions are important to finding the perfect blend of cosmetics for your skin.

FRAME IT

Frame your face with a hairstyle that fits its shape.

The shape of my face is:

    OVAL   RECTANGULAR   SQUARE   ROUND   HEART

FIX IT

Whether you want to fix the style or restore its shape, the right products will do wonders for your hair.

My hair is

    DRY   OILY   DULL   STRAIGHT   CURLY   FINE   COARSE

To avoid frustration, find a hairstyle that will easily work with the texture of your hair.

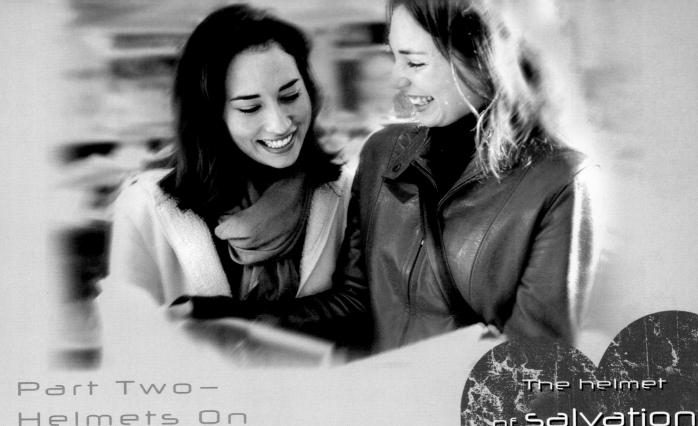

Part Two—
Helmets On

The helmet of **salvation** prevents us from losing our heads.

Knowledge is power. And knowing that you are saved through a relationship with Jesus Christ affects what you say and how you behave. Understanding who you are as a Christian unleashes power and persuasion that Satan would like to squelch. He'd love to get into your head and change your mind about God and your relationship to him. As Christians it's important that we keep our minds protected from Satan's mind games. ✳ Although the other pieces of armor are needed to sustain us, the helmet of salvation helps us see how they all relate. Without the knowledge of salvation the rest of the armor would be worn in vain. We love and commit to God with our hearts. But to avoid the devil's tricks, we need to use our head knowledge to drive us physically and intellectually.

Have you ever said or done something you wished you hadn't? Have you ever lost your head? I have. I felt like a brief moment of insanity took over my brain and I totally lost control of my thinking. I allowed Satan to feed my thoughts, and the results were terrible. I didn't have my helmet secure, and I fell right into the enemy's trap.

Ephesians 6:17—Take the helmet of salvation. . . .

When you were younger did your teacher ever say, "It's time to put our thinking caps on"? Everyone in the class would take out their invisible thinking caps and physically go through the motions of putting them on and tying them tight so they were ready to think. Do you think this

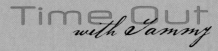

My son, Matthew, had a motorized scooter that he rode to work. One day when he was running late, he raced around looking for his helmet, found it, threw it on top of his head, and sped off down the street. Moments later my neighbor knocked on the door and asked me to come quickly. He had Matthew sprawled out in his car, head bleeding and only semiconscious. He had found him lying on the side of the road with his scooter and helmet a few feet away from him.

I took him directly to the hospital, where they ran tests and x-rays. They determined that besides the visible cuts and bruises, Matt had suffered a concussion. Once he started to come around and was alert enough to answer questions, the doctor came in to fill out the accident report. He asked, "Your mom says you were wearing a helmet, but I don't understand how you scraped up the top of your head?" "Well, I was wearing a helmet, but...," Matt confessed, "I didn't have it fastened." With that the doctor flew into a tailspin and told him how lucky he was to be alive.

Matt learned a tough lesson that day, not only about taking time to be responsible but also about how our lives are affected for good or bad by the way we process our thoughts. Matt's thought process went something like this: "I've driven this scooter dozens of times and nothing has ever happened, so what are the chances that I'm going to have an accident today and wish I'd buckled my helmet?" Matthew knew what could happen if he didn't wear his helmet the proper way, yet he still chose to only put it halfway on. He laid it on top of his head but he didn't fasten the strap.

How many of us are like that in our relationship with the Lord? We have the information we need to make wise decisions laying on top of our heads, but we haven't secured it to our minds. Like Matt, we figure we've been safe thus far, so why worry? I'll tell you why: Because Satan is just waiting to catch you off guard. So don't forget to fasten your salvation helmet; take the knowledge of it and apply it to your life!

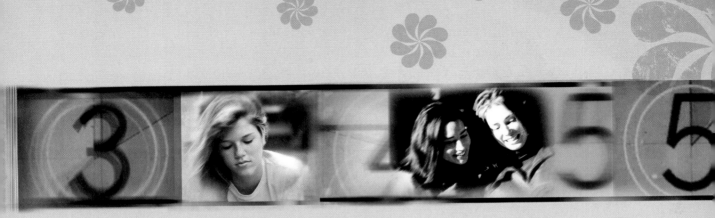

make-believe hat helped? It didn't make you any smarter, but it did focus your attention on what was coming up next. The action of putting it on made you stop, think, and become aware.

Well, in order for the helmet of salvation to do its job, you have to put it on and fasten it into place, just like those thinking caps.

Soulful Solutions

Satan's number one goal, whether you are a believer or not, is to make you doubt God. If you already know God, Satan will work at making you uncertain about God so he can hinder your spiritual growth and make you ineffective as God's witness. If you don't know God personally, Satan will continue filling your head with doubts so he can keep you from having a relationship with God.

Remember the story of Sleeping Beauty? When she was an infant, her parents, the king and queen, gave her away in order to protect her. Even though her parents didn't raise her, she didn't live in a palace, and she didn't even know who she really was, she was still a princess by bloodline. Nothing could change the fact that Aurora was the daughter of a king.

Well, guess what? If you've accepted Jesus Christ as your Lord and Savior, you're covered by his blood, and you are the daughter of the King—a princess. No one can take that away from you. As a daughter of the King, you must never doubt who you are.

Romans 8:17—Now if we are children, then we are heirs—heirs of God and co-heirs with Christ. . . .

Every time you make a mistake Satan will tell you that you're not good enough to belong to Christ. But don't believe him for a split second. It's Satan's goal to nag at you over and over again until you're not sure who you are anymore. Once you question your position in Christ, you become ineffective in your witness for him.

Sin hinders your spiritual growth and distances your relationship with God, but there's nothing you can do that will make him disown you. Put your thinking cap on, tie it up tight, and remember this: When you do something wrong, no matter how big or small, and your relationship with God needs restoration, ask forgiveness and he will forgive you. God doesn't hold grudges, no matter what Satan tries to make you think.

Scripture It

Roman soldiers wore helmets for the same reasons we do today—to protect their heads from blows that could injure or kill. Our heads contain our brains, the center of our thoughts, words, and actions. So if the enemy can successfully manipulate your head, he can really injure you. He'll maneuver your mouth and actions, and he'll try to make you a puppet in his hands.

Thought

All sin begins with one single thought.

Proverbs 4:23 (CEV)—Carefully guard your thoughts because they are the source of true life.

Satan distracts us and feeds our thoughts in numerous ways. Music, movies, television, videos, Internet—these things make it hard to keep our minds focused on God. Although difficult, we can keep our focus, even in the hardest of circumstances. Here's a little tip. If Satan gets to you through the music you listen to, things you watch, or Internet sites you visit, then take a deep breath and reach over and **turn them off.** It can take great willpower and drastic measures to turn off what Satan's turned you on to, but if you sincerely are seeking change, you can do it.

Talk

Think before you speak.

If Satan can feed our thoughts, he can affect our words and how we use them. Satan often holds your thoughts captive where your parents are concerned. He wants nothing more than to strain that relationship, and he'll stop at nothing to destroy it. His most common mode of operation is to manipulate your mind so that you disrespect your parents in the way you talk to them or by not talking to them at all.

Parents (me included) want to protect you from making the same mistakes we made when we were your age. Our parents did it to us, and believe it or not, a few years down the road you'll be doing it to your teens too. Be patient with your parents; they are human and will make mistakes. But you will too. Do the grown-up thing and discuss your difference of opinion. Your parents may not always agree with you, but they will respect your maturity.

Proverbs 6:20–23 (MESSAGE)—Good friend, follow your father's good advice; don't wander off from your mother's teachings. Wrap yourself in them from head to foot; wear them like a scarf around your neck. Wherever you walk, they'll guide you; wherever you rest, they'll guard you; when you wake up, they'll tell you what's next. For sound advice is a beacon, good teaching is a light, moral discipline is a life path.

Have you ever opened your mouth and said something about someone that you wish you hadn't? Satan loves to attack our words by tempting us to gossip. The glamour and glory that accompany being "in the know" intensify the excitement of "being the one to tell." There's a rush of power and popularity that overcomes us when we divulge a juicy piece of gossip, whether or not it's true. But when we are the one having gossip repeated about us we feel helpless and just look for a way to escape the torment. Gossip brings grief and destroys relationships.

Proverbs 16:28 (MESSAGE)—Troublemakers start fights; gossips break up friendships.

Walk

Think twice about the consequences of your actions.

It's important to weigh the cost of what you do. I know there are risks attached to everything you do, but we both know some things contain greater risks than others. Going to school, the hair salon, or the mall contains risks, but they are minimal compared to the risks of parties, dating, and hanging out with the wrong people. All too often, we put ourselves into predicaments that produce bigger consequences than we are prepared to deal with.

Satan wants the wrong decisions in a teen's life to look like "no brainers." He plants thoughts in your head like "Just go to the party, you want to be cool, don't you? Everyone will be there." These mind games are challenging, and Satan's next trick is to convince you that you can go to the party without being negatively affected. Once he gets you to the party, Satan moves to plan B. He says, "Go ahead, what's one little sip of beer going to hurt? You want to fit in, don't you?" The next thing you know, one sip turns into two, two into three . . . and there goes the first bottle.

Satan is tricky. He's too cunning for you and me to deal with alone; our minds are no match for his scheming. We need God's help to make sound decisions. I've said it before, but allow me to emphasize it again; spiritual maturity is key to battling the enemy. Cultivating your relationship with Jesus Christ through Bible reading and prayer helps you to keep walking in him.

When **doubt** comes about, pull your testimony out.

Colossians 2:6–8 (CEV)—You have accepted Christ Jesus as your Lord. Now keep on following him. Plant your roots in Christ and let him be the foundation for your life. Be strong in your faith, just as you were taught. And be grateful. Don't let anyone fool you by using senseless arguments. These arguments may sound wise, but they are only human teachings. They come from the powers of the world and not from Christ.

Satan will try to make you doubt your relationship with God. He'll work at this in a variety of ways, from planting seeds of uncertainty (like when you study Darwin's theory in school) to making you think that you're not worthy of God's love because you've messed up. He'll explore every avenue and try to find one that works on you. So be prepared. Know your testimony; write down your personal story of how you came to know Jesus Christ as your Lord and Savior. Sign it, date it, and put it in a prominent place to be looked at whenever the enemy strikes you with flashes of skepticism.

You can use this space to record your testimony. Don't worry about spelling and grammar. This is for your eyes only.

❋ What This Means 2U

Romans 12:2 (CEV)—Don't be like the people of this world, but let God change the way you think. Then you will know how to do everything that is good and pleasing to him.

In the blink of an eye, our thoughts can go from productive to destructive. So stay aware of your thinking. Commit your thinking to the Lord every day. Keep your helmet positioned and ready for battle at a moment's notice.

Thinking straight is a continual struggle. It sounds easy enough, but it's more difficult than it sounds. I don't know how often I'll be driving down the road, thinking to myself about one thing or another, and then all of a sudden I realize that I'm thinking about something totally ridiculous. Guard your mind with prayer and Bible study so you can stay alert and God-focused.

❧Test It Out

Don't let Satan capture you off guard. If you find yourself thinking about something you shouldn't, quickly pray and ask God to forgive you and change your thoughts. The next time you're listening to music, pay attention to where your thoughts are. The next time you watch television or a movie, be aware of what you're thinking. Judge for yourself whether the situation is putting you in a healthy state of mind. Always think about what you're thinking about!

Secure your thoughts in the knowledge of God's Word.

Ask God to change your thoughts when they get off track.

Listen to how you talk to your parents. Is it respectful?

View your testimony often in order to detour doubt.

Aim your focus on the things of God.

Take your thoughts captive.

Increase awareness of what you are thinking.

Occupy your mind with the things of God.

Never open your mind to outside influences (hypnosis, trances, alcohol, drugs).

Super Models have the **heads up** on thinking.

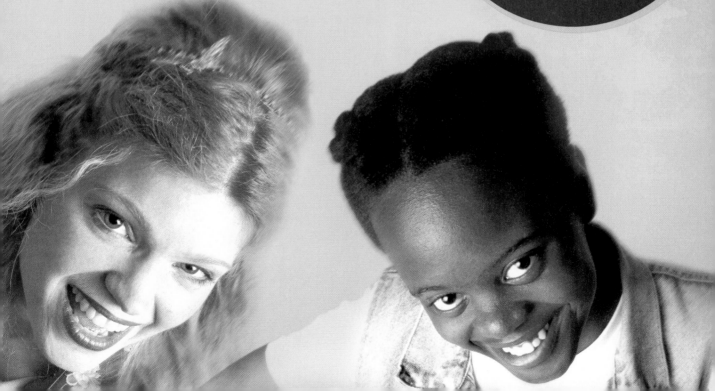

It's in the Bag

Part One—
Purse with Purpose

Purses, handbags, totes, and backpacks—finding the perfect pouch to meet your needs and match your personal style is worth the effort. Bags are fun because they come in a variety of styles and colors. But they're also functional, designed to carry everything from a laptop to a lipstick. The way you carry your personal things is your choice; the possibilities are only limited by personal preference and imagination. ✳ Have you ever played the packing game? "I'm going on a trip and I'm going to take such-and-such with me . . ." In this chapter, we're going to learn how to pack for both daily routines and special occasions. We'll learn what we should have and must have in our pocketbooks or book bags. So get ready to dump out your purse, backpack, or gym bag, and we'll repack it according to your needs.

Picking a purse with purpose, a happening handbag, or a sensible satchel can be confusing when we're not sure what we need or want. I'm drawn to cute little evening bags that couldn't carry my wallet even if I cut it in half. Although they are just right for going out on the town, toting a lipstick and tissue, they don't meet my needs for everyday use. What I am drawn to and what I need are two totally different things. But I've learned to balance the two so I still tote my stuff in style.

What's in your purse? If you're like me, it's good to clean it out and reorganize it every once in awhile so you can lighten the load and restock what you're running out of. Our purses and their contents are as unique as our personalities, but we all need to transport our goods. Whether it's by backpack, pocket, or sock, having necessities on hand makes life easier.

> Change purses and changing purses are both fun and **functional.**

✳ Simple Solutions

Everyone seems to want something different. Some gals carry around purses the size of small suitcases, while others stick things in their pockets and don't carry a purse at all. The trick is to balance what you must have with you with the kind of purse, pocket, or satchel you want. In my case, I want a purse that is practical yet cute. With a little know-how, it's possible to have it all.

The first step to finding a well-matched bag for your stuff is to know what you want to carry with you. If you're carrying everything but the kitchen sink, you'll need a huge bag, but if you're only carrying a few bucks and an identification card, you can make due with a miniorganizer. Use the information below to determine what you want or need to carry with you.

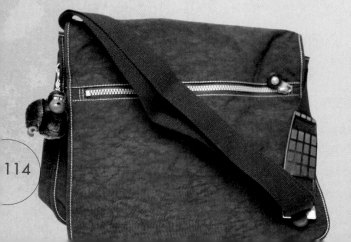

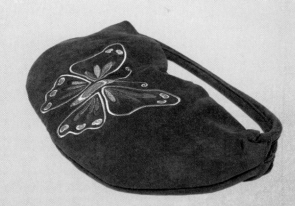

Wallet

- Money
- Identification Card
- License
- Pictures
- Loose Change
- Safety Pins
- Band-Aids
- Color Swatches (see page 12)
- Receipts

Cosmetic or Ziploc Bag

- Powder Compact with Mirror
- Zit Cream (to dry blemishes)
- Concealer (to touch up blemishes)
- Blush
- Retractable Makeup Brush
- Lip Liner
- Lip Color
- Hand Cream
- Nail Glue
- Nail File
- Travel-Size Deodorant
- Comb/Brush
- Travel-Size Hairspray
- Perfume (Sample Size)
- Ponytail Holder/Barrette
- Travel-Size Sunscreen

Emergency

- Cell Phone
- Emergency Phone Numbers
- Sanitary Pad/Tampon
- Aspirin (check school policy)
- Prescription Medicines (check school policy)
- Glasses/Case
- Contact Lenses Case

Miscellaneous

- Keys
- Coin Purse
- Pen/Pencil
- Paper
- Travel Umbrella
- Breath Mints
- Gum
- Tissues
- Small Flashlight
- Eyeglass Repair Kit
- Calendar/Assignment Book
- Travel Toothbrush/Toothpaste
- Wax for Braces
- Disposable Camera
- Travel Bible
- Calculator
- Pocket Dictionary
- Business Cards (ex: Babysitting)
- Travel Sewing Kit
- Travel Lint Remover
- Other

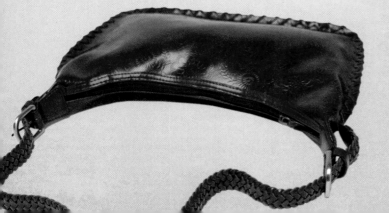

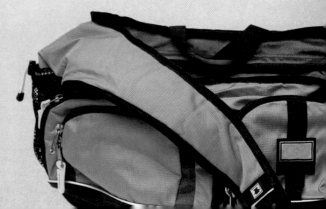

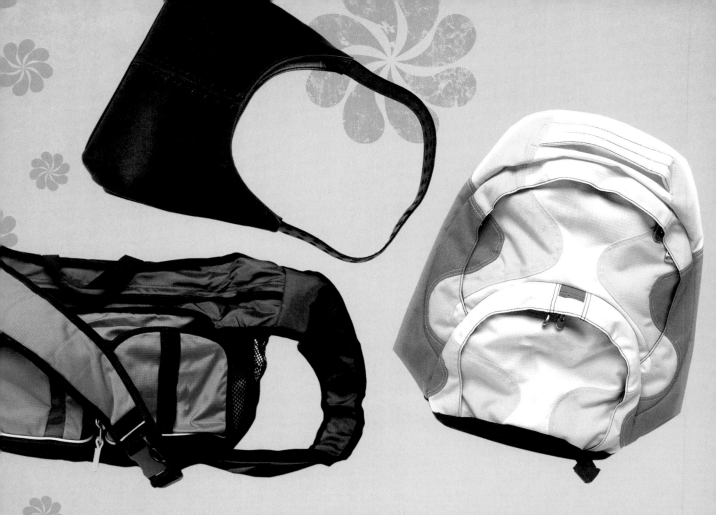

Wow, what a list! Did you ever think you needed so much stuff? I bet you have things on your list I never thought of. I'm amazed at what people carry in their purses. I have one friend who carries tea bags and another who keeps all-occasion cards just in case she suddenly remembers a birthday or anniversary. The fact is, we all have stuff—whether a little or a lot—and we need a way to transport it.

Look over your list. How many items have you checked off? Will you need a small, medium, or large bag? Not sure? Then read on.

PICTURE IT

With so many choices at your fingertips, it's best to narrow your selection by determining what size bag you're going to need before you get started: small, medium, or large. Next, consider what shape and style of bag you're interested in. It's nice to start off with a basic, everyday purse to accompany you just about anywhere.

To help narrow your choices, you should also consider what color leather shoes and belt you typically wear—black or brown. I normally wear black because black is a member of the cool color family, while brown is a member of the warm color family. You don't *have* to match your leathers to your skin tone because they don't come in contact with your face, but a matching leather will blend better with the colors in your wardrobe.

Below you will find a list of handbags to familiarize yourself with. Take this list to a store and ask the clerk to show you examples of the various styles and fabrics. Still baffled? For more handbag insight visit www.ebags.com.

Shapes and Styles

- Zip-Top Shoulder
- Backpack
- Bowling Bag
- Double Handled
- Drawstring
- Flap
- Hobo
- Messenger/Courier Bag
- Mini Bag
- Mini Backpack
- Duffle
- Multicompartment
- Organizer
- Satchel
- Short Shoulder
- Wristlet Handle
- Briefcase Bag
- Sling
- Tote/Carry All
- Evening
- Pouch (no handle)
- Double-Handled Box Bag

Common Closures

- Drawstring
- Snap
- Zipper
- Buckle
- Velcro
- Flap

Handy Handles

- Chain Shoulder Strap
- Bauble Handle
- Rope Handle
- Padded
- Bamboo

Fabulous Fabrics

- Canvas
- Denim
- Linen
- Leather
- Vinyl
- Nylon/Micro Fiber
- Plaids/Checks
- Quilted
- Tapestry
- Faux Fur
- Woven
- Beaded
- Silk
- Satin
- Embroidery
- Tassel/Fringe
- Sequined
- Lace
- Pearls
- Ribbon
- Crochet
- Straw

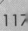

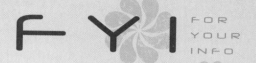

> There's one more thing to consider when choosing the perfect handbag. Pick one that complements your size. If you are petite, carrying a huge purse will look off balance, and if you are tall, carrying a handbag with a short shoulder strap will make you look even taller. So remember to pick a purse that's sized just for you.

✳ What This Means 2U

It doesn't matter if your handbag is for everyday use, or if you bought it to complement a specific outfit; as a fashion accessory, it serves an extremely important purpose.

I could go without a belt or earrings and be fine, but when I forget my pocketbook I go into purse panic. Someone once told me that if she lost her purse, she'd lose her identity because it contained everything from her driver's license to her diary. I don't know what it is, but there's something about a girl and her purse. It's our own personal space, and we don't want anyone rummaging through it. So whether you carry a pocketbook or backpack, it's more than just an accessory—it's your accomplice.

❧ Test It Out

You can tell a lot about someone's personal style by their purse. Do you dump everything into a hobo sack and rummage through it to find what you're looking for? Or do you have a courier bag so you can carry your books and always be ready to work? Whatever your style, purses are important. They carry some of our most prized possessions, so carefully consider what it is you'll be toting with you. Buy a purse with purpose to match your size and style.

PACK IT

Review your packing list on page 115. Is your list short, long, or somewhere in between?

How many items are on your list?

How many items are small, such as pencils, pens, or lipstick?

Will these items require their own pocket or compartment?

    YES   NO

How many items are medium sized, such as a cell phone or coin purse?

Would you prefer to have these items in their own separate compartments for easy accessibility?

    YES   NO

How many items are large, such as a wallet, cosmetic bag, or assignment book?

Will these items require a bag of any special shape or size?

    YES   NO

PICK IT

Do you consider your body shape or frame to be:

SMALL   MEDIUM   LARGE

What about your height?

SHORT   AVERAGE   TALL

What is your body shape?

Pear   Rectangle   Apple   Hourglass   Wedge

Here are some handbag suggestions based on your size and shape.

That's My Bag

Shape	Frame		Height	
	Small to Medium	Medium to Large	Short to Average	Average to Tall
Pear	Satchel	Backpack	Short shoulder hobo	Sling
Rectangle	Organizer	Bowling Bag	Flap	Courier
Apple	Small tote	Drawstring	Multi-compartment	Hobo
Hourglass	Backpack	Drawstring Sling	Short shoulder hobo	Hobo
Wedge	Sling	Bowling Bag	Satchel	Duffle

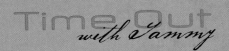

Time Out
with Tammy

My daughter, Ashlee, is quite petite and weighs around a hundred pounds. Once she entered high school she started having back problems due to the weight of her backpack.

She had to carry all her books in her backpack around campus because her high school did not have lockers. When I took her to the doctor to have her back examined, she happened to have her book bag with her, and when the nurse weighed the bag, it was thirty-two pounds! Ashlee had been toting almost a third of her body weight, and the doctor informed us that she shouldn't be carrying more than ten percent of her weight.

Knowing Ashlee could develop serious health problems, the doctor sent a letter to the school stating the obvious; Ashlee's backpack was causing her back problems. Not only was it too heavy for her, but it also caused her to hunch over, creating poor posture. Although it took a somewhat drastic measure, the school resolved the problem by supplying Ashlee with two sets of books, one set for home use and one for school.

If your backpack is causing back problems, check to make sure you're carrying no more than ten percent of your body weight. Always wear both straps (the wider the better), and if the problem persists, talk to the school. Even if the pain is minor now, it has the potential to cause severe damage in the future. Be good to your body and it will serve you well.

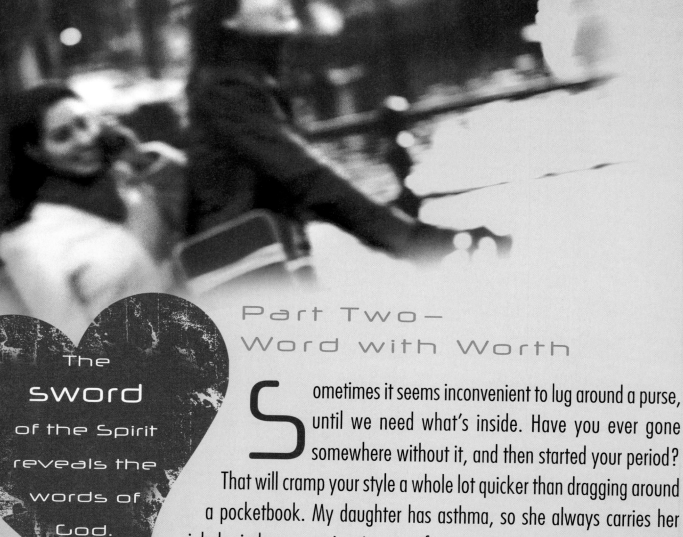

Part Two—
Word with Worth

The **sword** of the Spirit reveals the words of God.

Sometimes it seems inconvenient to lug around a purse, until we need what's inside. Have you ever gone somewhere without it, and then started your period? That will cramp your style a whole lot quicker than dragging around a pocketbook. My daughter has asthma, so she always carries her inhaler in her purse, just in case of an emergency. Carrying a bag with you, whether or not you need it, can give you peace of mind. ❋ I've even heard of girls using their purse as an offensive weapon to beat off attackers. The armor of God also includes an offensive weapon that you should carry for protection at all times—the sword of the Spirit, which is the Word of God. So far we've dressed to defend ourselves against the enemy. Now it's time to take up the only offensive part. In it you will find both practical and protective help for anything you'll ever need.

Have you ever had a hard time making a decision? Have you ever hunted for answers to problems that seemed impossible to solve? Maybe you've wondered about the truth concerning sex, dating, or homosexuality. Or maybe you've contemplated what kind of guy you should marry. In all of these cases, it can be difficult to sort out right from wrong.

Well, guess what? You can receive insight to all of life's questions if you just look in the right spot.

2 Timothy 3:16–17 (MESSAGE)—Every part of Scripture is God-breathed and useful one way or another—showing us truth, exposing our rebellion, correcting our mistakes, training us to live God's way. Through the Word we are put together and shaped up for the tasks God has for us.

Soulful Solutions

Ephesians 6:17—Take the . . . sword of the Spirit, which is the Word of God.

The Bible says *"take"* the sword, which literally means to get possession of it; to obtain it. The soldier's sword was used for hand-to-hand combat. Although the other pieces of the armor were extremely important, the sword was the only offensive weapon the soldier had readily available in the event of an unexpected attack. The soldier's sword was made of iron, it was usually around twenty-four inches long, it was sharpened on both sides (double-edged), and it hung in a leather sheath from his belt so that it could be drawn in a moment.

So, why is the Bible called the sword of the Spirit? Well, God's Word has an answer for everything, so let's look there for an answer to this question. Here's how to do it:

1. Know the topic of interest or key words.

2. Look up the topic or key words in your Bible's concordance (a concordance is an alphabetical list of words, with references to the passages in which they occur). If your Bible doesn't have a concordance, refer to a separate concordance (found in your church library or Christian bookstore).

3. Narrow down the answer by looking up the verses which refer to the topic or key words.

It's that simple. So let's get started with our question: Why is the Bible referred to as the sword of the Spirit?

1. The key word here is *sword*.

2. Look up the word *sword* in your Bible's concordance.

3. Read the passages of Scripture that make reference to the word *sword* in order to narrow down your choices and find the answer.

My concordance listed several passages of Scripture for the word *sword*, but after reading through them I was able to narrow the answer down to this verse in the Book of Hebrews.

Hebrews 4:12 (NKJV)—For the word of God is living and powerful, and sharper than any two-edged sword, piercing even to the division of soul and spirit, and of joints and marrow, and is a discerner of the thoughts and intents of the heart.

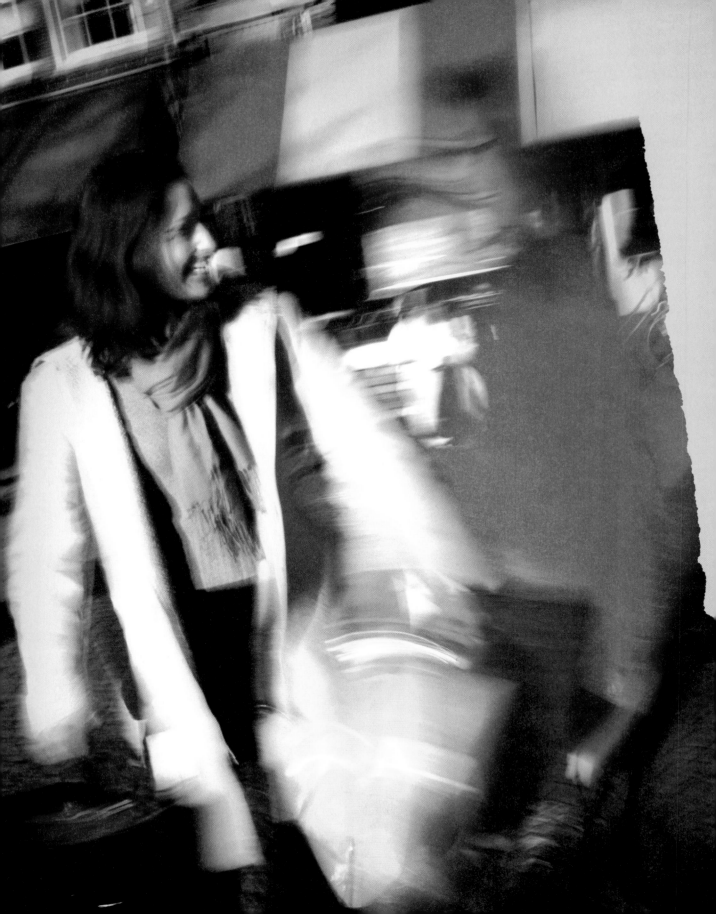

The Bible is called a sword because it cuts down to who we really are, both good and bad. With it, we can know God, discern right from wrong, and shape our lives according to God's plan for our lives. God's Word is living and powerful. In it you will find answers to life's most difficult questions.

Scripture It

The Bible, like no other book, is unique in the fact that it's either 100 percent true, or 100 percent false. You cannot say, "I believe this, but not that." It's all or nothing. If you doubt even one word, the whole Bible becomes questionable.

There may be things that you don't understand in the Bible, and that's normal. It's when you question the Bible's credibility that it becomes an issue of truth. There are many things that my feeble mind can't comprehend; yet I never question the validity of Scripture.

Satan tries to use this lack of understanding against us. Did you know that Satan quoted Scripture when he tempted Jesus? In Luke 4, Satan appears before Jesus when he is at a physically weak point. Then Satan misrepresents the Scripture, hoping that Jesus will misunderstand the Word of God.

> Luke 4:9–12—The devil led him to Jerusalem and had him stand on the highest point of the temple. "If you are the Son of God," he said, "throw yourself down from here. For it is written: 'He will command his angels concerning you to guard you carefully; they will lift you up in their hands, so that you will not strike your foot against a stone.'" Jesus answered, "It says: 'Do not put the Lord your God to the test.'"

How's that for gutsy? Satan attempted to twist Scripture that was inspired by God and use it against him. Although he quoted it perfectly, he took it out of context. (Read Psalm 91 in its entirety and you'll see what I mean.) He picked a couple verses from Psalms and ignored the rest of Scripture so that it would suit his purposes.

Luckily for us, the crafty devil is no match for our God. As hard as Satan tried to put a spin on Scripture and ruin Christ, Jesus just turned around and threw the truth of God's Word right back in his face. He used the sword of the Spirit in hand-to-hand combat against the devil.

Each of us is faced with different issues and challenges that we must be prepared for. Some are larger than others, but we must be equipped to handle whatever comes our way. Just like packing our purses with the things we need, we must pack our brains with knowledge of the Bible so we're ready with what we need at a moment's notice. We must learn to test temptations against the truth of the Scriptures so that we can live well-balanced lives. So when Satan tempts you, have your sword ready!

I know what you are thinking, "How can I possibly carry my Bible and have it ready 24/7?" Well, it's nice to have a little pocket Bible in your purse, but it's what you pack in your brain that really matters. It's all about studying and memorizing Bible verses.

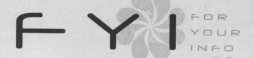

Studying and memorizing Bible verses isn't as hard as it sounds. I'm living proof; because if I can do it, anyone else can memorize too. A wise man once told me that memorization is nothing more than determination. If you think you can, you will; and if you think you can't, you won't. It's that simple. So trust me, Bible memorization isn't just another homework assignment. Long after you've forgotten algebra, you'll be able to recall a Bible verse just exactly when you need it.

Psalm 119:11—I have hidden your word in my heart that I might not sin against you.

The first step to memorization is finding a method that works for you. Do you learn by sight? Do you learn audibly? Do you learn best hands-on? Or are you like me and learn a little of each way? Below you will find some ideas for Scripture memorization. Pick the methods that suit you best.

Sing the verse. Buy a children's CD of compiled verses put to song. This is a fun and easy way to learn verses.

Write the verse. I know someone who writes verses on small cards and then tapes them to the dashboard of his car so he can memorize while he's stuck in traffic.

Say it out loud. Recite the verse over and over again out loud to yourself or a friend until you get it.

Make memorizing a game. Set memorizing goals and then reward yourself when you meet the challenge. You could even challenge your friends or siblings to a contest.

Erase a word. Use a small size dry-erase board to write the verse on. Then read it and practice reciting it. Next erase a few words and say it again. Repeat this process until the verse has been totally erased.

Exercise it. Exercising is a great time to memorize verses. I'll jot down a verse on a card or print it off on the computer and then take it with me when I'm walking. This is a great way to take your mind off of exercise and onto God.

Verse calendar. Use your computer and make a calendar with a verse or verses to memorize during each month or week. Hang it in a prominent spot in your room.

These are just a few ideas to get you started. In time, you'll find the one that works best for you. You may even think up some clever ways to memorize on your own.

Is there anything that you personally struggle with? Anger, alcohol, disrespect, drugs, sex, stealing, lying, cheating, etc.? Find a verse to combat the sin, read it, write it, and memorize it. I struggle with being too busy to spend time alone with God. The verse that I memorized, framed, and place throughout my home is:

Psalm 46:10—Be still, and know that I am God. . . .

Whenever I think there is no time, I stop to reflect on this verse and put things into their proper perspective. Then I make the time.

Write the reference and verse that you want to memorize below:

❋ What This Means 2U

I'd like to share with you what someone shared with me during the summer I spent in Mexico. It's probably the best description of the Bible I've ever read. In fact, I wrote it in the front cover of my Bible.

The Bible

This book contains the mind of God, the state of man, the way of salvation, the doom of sinners, and the happiness of believers.

Its doctrines are holy, its precepts are binding, its histories are true, and its decisions immutable.

Read it to be wise, believe it to be safe, and practice it to be holy.

It contains light to direct you, food to support you, and comfort to cheer you.

It is the traveler's map, the pilgrim's staff, the pilot's compass, the soldier's sword, and the Christian's character.

Here paradise is restored, heaven opened, and the gates of hell disclosed.

Christ is its grand subject, our good its design, and the glory of God its end.

It should fill the memory, rule the heart, and guide the feet.

Read it slowly, frequently, and prayerfully.

It is a mine of wealth, a paradise of glory, and a river of pleasure.

Follow its precepts and it will lead you to Calvary, to the empty tomb, to resurrected life in Christ, and yes, to glory itself, for all eternity.

~ Author Unknown

Matthew 24:35 (CEV)—The sky and the earth won't last forever, but my words will.

❧ Test It Out

Like Jesus, be ready with the Word when Satan tempts you. Ephesians 6:17 states, "Take the... sword of the Spirit, which is the Word of God." Since it's virtually impossible to take our Bibles with us everywhere, it's important that we know what Scripture says, so we can take the truth with us wherever we go.

Get into the habit of reading, studying, and memorizing Bible verses, and you'll find yourself ready whenever Satan comes knocking at your door. You can attack him with the truth of God's Word when he tries to get you off track. So whether you're packing your book bag or your brain, always be prepared.

Stand firm on the promises of the Bible.

Worship God through his Word (Psalm 118:24).

Obligate yourself to spend at least ten minutes a day reading the Bible.

Reflect on the Word of God often.

Determine to memorize Scripture.

Super Models draw the **SWORD** of the Spirit.

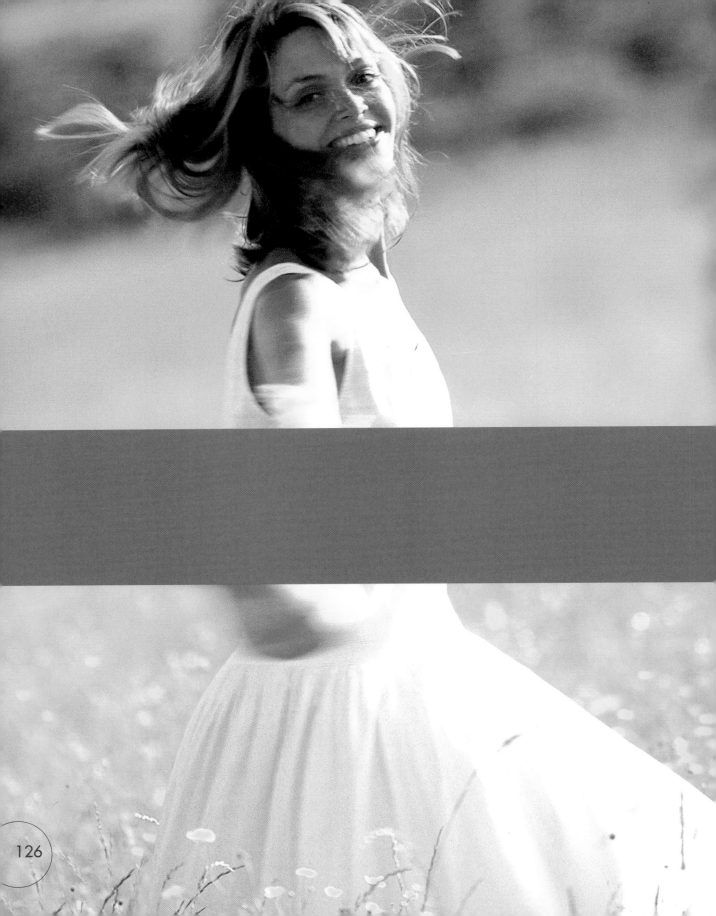

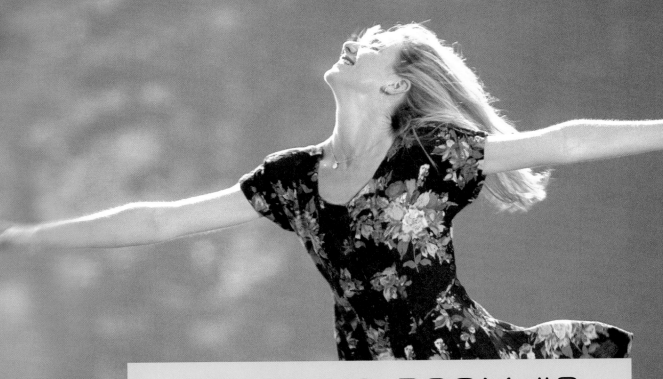

Chick Chat

Part One—Girl Talk

On a scale from one to ten, how would you rate your sense of style? Are you a one who needs major help, or a ten who's got it all together? Or are you like the majority of women, who lie somewhere in between, looking for a way to cut through the hype and find sound advice on self-image? ✳ We're going to look at what it takes to be a Super Model, and we'll also learn where self-image comes from and how it affects every area of our lives. Read on, and in just a few moments you'll know

how to improve your appearance, act self-confident, and feel good about yourself from the inside out.

I phoned one of the top modeling agencies in the world and asked, "What is the number one quality a girl must possess to be a super model?" To my surprise, it wasn't healthy hair, a flawless face, a perfectly proportioned figure, or long legs; it was faith! You must have faith in yourself to enter the harsh modeling world, possessing an endless supply of self-confidence.

Wow! That answer blew me away. I've had a taste of both modeling and acting, but self-confidence never entered my mind when I thought about finding success in the business. However, it makes sense that you must possess this important attribute in order to survive the seemingly endless rejection that comes with either occupation. It's known as having *thick skin*—you can handle rejection because you're secure in yourself.

In the next few pages I'm going to help you put on the most important item a Super Model wears, and that's faith in herself.

The very first step to becoming a Super Model of any kind is to like yourself. You must like who you are if you expect others to like you too. If you like yourself—by being confident but not conceited—your positive attitude will show from the inside out, and others will be attracted to you. If you don't like yourself and you put yourself down, others will either join in the putdowns or just avoid you and your downer attitude.

You are a role model to someone. But what type of role are you? Is your role an act or is the *real* you on display? Do people really know *you*, or have they met an imitation of someone else you're trying to be? These are really tough questions. God created us to feel, and as a result we often build invisible barriers around who we are in order to guard ourselves from rejection. Before we go any further, take a minute and judge for yourself; who are you on the inside? Only you can honestly answer that question.

Describe who you are on the inside:

Describe how others see you on the outside:

What's the difference between the two?

Which person do you like better—the person you are on the outside or the person you are on the inside? Why?

Improving your **self-image** improves the way you look and feel.

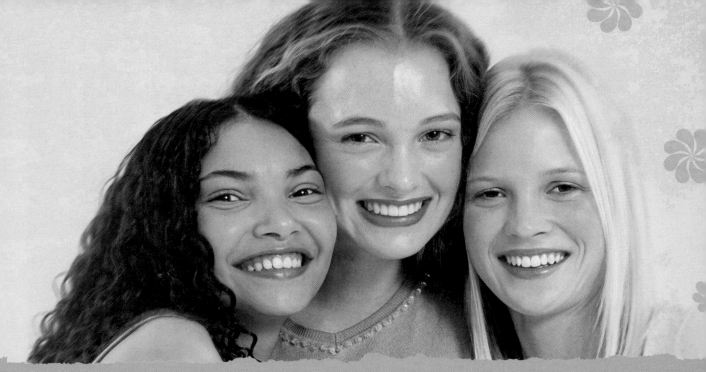

Have you ever felt like you have a split personality because you act one way around one group of friends, another way around a different group of friends, and yet another way at home? During my teenage years I had friends at school, church friends, and my family to contend with, and these were three very different roles.

Tammy with her friends at school: "Hey, are you going to the party after Friday's game? It cracks me up to watch what's-his-face get wasted."

Tammy with her church friends: "I'd never go to a party where there are drugs and alcohol present."

Tammy at home: "Don't worry, I don't drink or do drugs and there won't be any of those things at the party…and yes, the parents will be home."

In reality I was a little bit of each role, but I didn't fit into any one whole role. I love being surrounded by people, so Tammy #1 went to parties, but I didn't like the drinking and drugs that were there. However, I'd usually carry a half-empty glass of beer around with me to give the appearance that I was drinking. Of course, going to those parties made Tammy #2 and #3 a big liar, something I didn't want to be. Although I didn't drink or use drugs, I did go to parties that damaged my credibility.

My basic problem was that I lacked self-esteem and had a poor self-image. I was afraid I'd be ridiculed if the real me spoke up and said, "Hey, everyone, party at my house Friday night; no drugs or alcohol allowed . . . and yes, my parents will be home!"

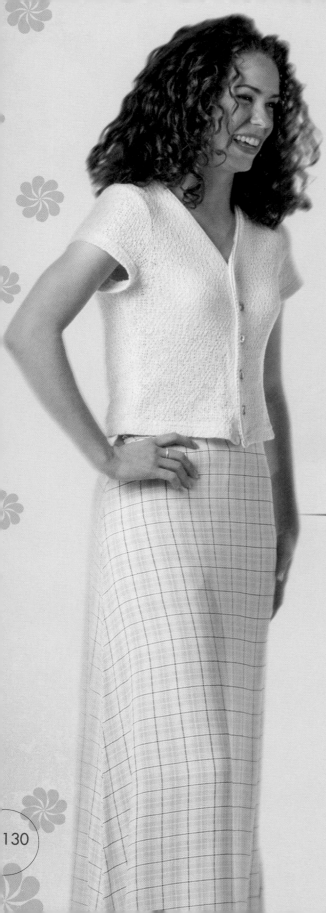

✳ Simple Solutions

Your self-esteem is made up of five fundamentals—the Physical, Emotional, Relational, Mental, and Spiritual. To shorten it, I'll just call these five fundamentals P.E.R.M.S.

I've had several perms over the years, and in order to get a good permanent there are five basic steps the stylist must complete:

1. Roll squeaky-clean shampooed hair in perm rods.
2. Apply perm solution and wait with watchful eye for the solution to do its thing.
3. Rinse well and blot dry.
4. Apply neutralizer and wait five minutes.
5. Remove perm rods and rinse thoroughly.

You must complete each step in order for the perm to work. My daughter once got a perm, and when the stylist didn't carefully follow the perm directions, my daughter's hair fell off. Luckily she was only having the ends permed or she would have been completely bald!

PICTURE IT 5

P.E.R.M.S., your physical, emotional, relational, mental, and spiritual status, are key to a healthy self-image. P.E.R.M.S. are self-esteem makeovers that look good on everybody. Just apply them well and you'll like who's looking back at you from the mirror.

Step #1—

Be All You Can Be Physically

Since we're so preoccupied with how we look on the outside, our physical state is a terrific place to start. When you look better, you feel better; and when you feel better, you act more confident. So take good care of your body.

Do's (good habits):

Practice good skin care.

Use makeup wisely.

Use a deodorant that works on you.

Floss and brush your teeth.

Be aware of bad breath; use a mouthwash, mints, or consult your dentist.

Wash your feet and use foot deodorant if you have a problem with stinky feet.

Wash your hair and keep it well-groomed.

Eat healthy and don't skip breakfast.

Drink noncarbonated beverages such as milk, juice, and water.

Get at least eight to ten hours of sleep per night, even on weekends.

Find an exercise you enjoy and do it.

Practice good posture. Sit and stand up straight; you'll not only feel better but you'll look better too.

Practice good etiquette; there's nothing wrong with saying "please" and "thank you."

Don'ts (bad habits):

Don't smoke cigarettes. Besides being extremely unhealthy, smoking costs big money, yellows your teeth, harms your skin, and makes your breath, hair, and clothes stink.

Don't drink alcoholic beverages. If you're a minor, it's illegal. Alcohol is bad for your skin, contributes to weight gain, leads to many diseases, and can impair your thinking, which leads to other disasters.

Don't use drugs, from marijuana to ecstasy. If you do use drugs or have a friend that does, find help.

Don't have sex to keep a boyfriend. Pressure is no reason to go all the way. Sex outside of marriage can harm you physically (STDs), but it can also destroy you emotionally and give you an unhealthy viewpoint on sex for the rest of your life.

Step #2—Be All You Can Be Emotionally

We easily get wrapped up in how we feel about something, but our feelings are often wrong. I remember feeling like a girl at school hated me, because the harder I tried to talk to her the more she seemed to avoid me. Finally, we got stuck together working on a biology project and I found out my feelings were wrong. She didn't hate me, she was just painfully shy. In fact, she was happy that I pursued the friendship.

Review the list below and circle the answers that best describe where you stand emotionally. Answer honestly.

Emotional Uppers Emotional Downers (1)—(a) My peers have a positive affect on me. (b) My peers affect me negatively. (2)—(a) I develop and maintain healthy friendships. (b) My friendships are unhealthy. (3)—(a) I set boundaries with my boyfriend. (b) I have no boundaries with my boyfriend. (4)—(a) I have a sound relationship with my parents. (b) I have a stressful relationship with my parents. (5)—(a) The TV/movies I watch give a positive influence. (b) The TV/movies I watch influence me in a negative way. (6)—(a) The music I listen to is fun and uplifting. (b) The music I listen to is demoralizing, destructive, and depressing. (7)—(a) My Internet usage is straight up. (b) I go to places on the Internet I don't want my parents to know about. (8)—(a) I practice good habits. (b) I've developed damaging habits (drugs, alcohol, cigarette smoking, etc.).

Emotional downers have a negative impact on your feelings. They affect your outlook on life, turning you into a "glass is half-empty" kind of person. When you are emotionally secure, your attitude changes for the better and so does your perspective.

Step #3—Be All You Can Be Relationally

Relationships with our family, friends, and peers influence us for the good or bad. Teen years in particular are shaped and molded by peer pressure. We're so desperate to fit in with our friends that we sacrifice our own self-image in order to be part of the group. Of the five areas that affect your self-worth, who you are relationally is by far the most influential, especially when it comes to peer pressure. So how can you battle negative peer pressure in a positive manner?

You must like yourself first. Believing in yourself—having faith in who you are as a Christian—is key to combating the ill effects of peer pressure.

And what about family? Sometimes it's just as difficult to be yourself at home as it is at school, especially when your family relationships are strained due to differences. I call this the square-peg-round-hole feeling, because it seems you just don't fit in no matter how you maneuver yourself. You feel as opposite from your parents as punk is from yuppie. And you wonder how on earth you ended up living with aliens. And you know what? Your parents are wondering the same thing.

I've been a teenager, and now I am the mom of teenagers. And I've learned that there's a growing process for both parties involved. When I was a teen, I had my own thoughts about my place in the world, and they didn't always jive with my parents' ideas. They wanted the best for me, just as I want what seems best for my teens. So show your parents you are maturing by being patient with them. Someday you'll want your teens to treat you the same way.

When it comes to relationships with family or friends, there's one more very important thing to address—abuse. Physical and mental abuse of any kind is wrong. It can have permanent, damaging effects if it's not dealt with. Always remember that you are not a bad person; the person who mistreats you is in the wrong. If you face an abusive situation, please get help. Find someone to tell, and if they don't listen to you, find someone who will. If you know someone who is experiencing abuse, be a friend and seek help for them.

Step #4—Be All You Can Be Mentally

Knowledge is power, so never stop learning. School is a requirement, but learning is a choice. Only you can choose to utilize your time well and apply yourself. I know school can be a drag, but your education is a great opportunity that many teens don't have.

When I was in high school my highest priority was socialization. I viewed education as some sort of yucky medicine that adults were forcing down my throat. My lack of interest in my high school education made it much more difficult for me to succeed later in life.

Enhance your self-image by setting goals that focus on the future. You had to crawl before you could walk, and you had to walk before you could run. Our goals are no different; we must master the small ones in order to reach the big ones, but achieving your goals requires effort on your part. For example, if you want to go to college later, you will have to pass algebra now.

Step #5—Be All You Can Be Spiritually

I've saved the best for last—your spiritual life. Who you are comes down to one basic question: Who are you in relationship to Jesus Christ? I've devoted more time to this topic than any other in the book and that's because everything else pales in comparison. When it's all over, there's only one thing that really matters in life: Did you take the time to know Jesus personally? If you're not sure, refer back to chapter 1.

Your soul is the source of purpose, significance, and inner peace. It's the most inward part that no one sees, but it drives your convictions, actions, and thoughts. Who are you spiritually? It's the most important question of life.

Faith lets you try, fear helps you fail.

❋ What This Means 2U
Self-confidence affects every area of your life. It can determine whether you get a D or a B in history, whether you attempt the goal in soccer, and whether you'll say no to a boyfriend who wants to score. "When you've failed to try, you've tried to fail," so the saying goes. Faith in God and in yourself enables you to try—and to succeed.

Super Models possess self-worth that allows them to focus on the goal, to never give up, to accept both their successes and their failures, and to keep on keepin' on. Remember, God loves you. Do you love yourself? And more importantly, do you like who you are and who you are becoming?

Test It Out

One of the most difficult relationships you can have is the one you have with yourself. It's often much easier to nurture and respect someone else. But God made you, and no matter what you might think, he doesn't make *any* mistakes. He created you to love him first, and to love your neighbor the same way you love yourself. This means you must love yourself in order to love others.

So take the time to get to know yourself. You might find out that there's a lot to like, and if there is anything you don't like, you have the power to change it. Faith in God and faith in one's self are key attributes to becoming a Super Model.

BE ALL YOU CAN BE PHYSICALLY

Put one good habit into practice this week: _____

Pledge to give up at least one bad habit: _____

BE ALL YOU CAN BE EMOTIONALLY

What changes can you make in your downer column to turn your emotions upward?

BE ALL YOU CAN BE RELATIONALLY

How do your friends affect who you are and what you do?
    Judging yourself as a peer, how do you affect others?

BE ALL YOU CAN BE MENTALLY

Where do you see yourself ten years from now?

Name one goal you can set to reach this ambition.

BE ALL YOU CAN BE SPIRITUALLY

How and when did you come to know Jesus personally?

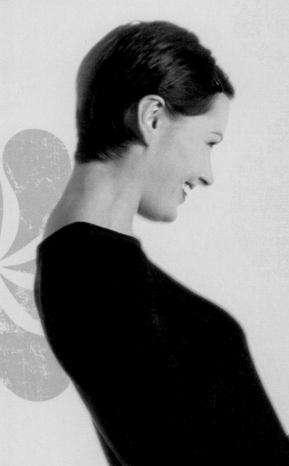

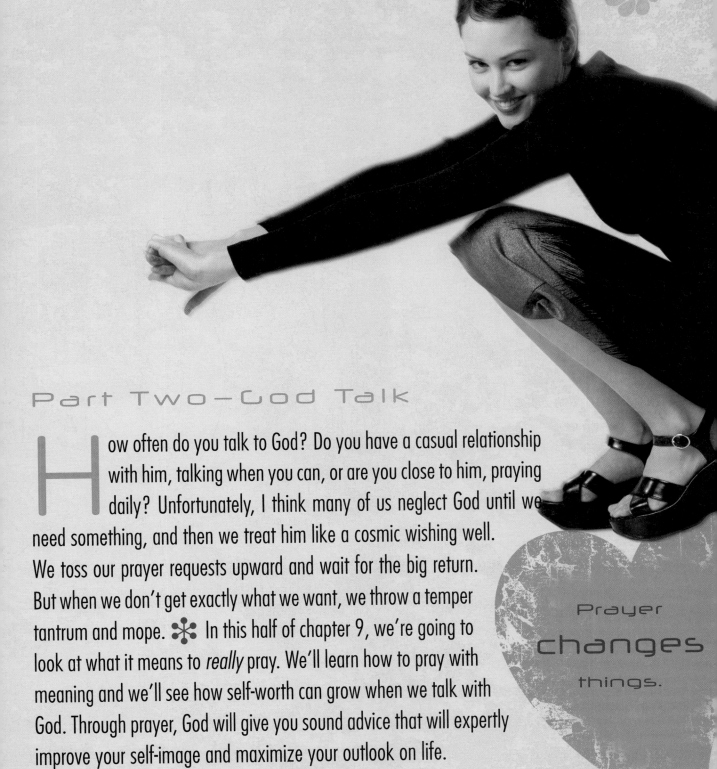

Part Two—God Talk

How often do you talk to God? Do you have a casual relationship with him, talking when you can, or are you close to him, praying daily? Unfortunately, I think many of us neglect God until we need something, and then we treat him like a cosmic wishing well. We toss our prayer requests upward and wait for the big return. But when we don't get exactly what we want, we throw a temper tantrum and mope. ❋ In this half of chapter 9, we're going to look at what it means to *really* pray. We'll learn how to pray with meaning and we'll see how self-worth can grow when we talk with God. Through prayer, God will give you sound advice that will expertly improve your self-image and maximize your outlook on life.

Prayer **changes** things.

Does God hear me? Why doesn't he answer? Why does he answer everyone else? What am I doing wrong?

Have you ever asked yourself any of those questions? I have. Over the years, I've discovered that lack of understanding hindered my communication with God. I thought I could just show up with my shopping list, rattle off what I wanted, and then cash out. I had no idea what it truly meant to pray. Once I realized the importance of prayer and learned how to pray, my relationship with God reached a new level. He truly became my best friend and confidant.

Do you have God's number? The call is toll-free, and the lines are open twenty-four hours a day, seven days a week. You'll never be put on hold or reach an annoying automated answering system. You'll talk to the Main Man himself, God your Father.

Although we often take this awesome privilege for granted, it's actually quite overwhelming when we put it in perspective. Think of it this way—when was the last time you picked up the phone and dialed up the President of the United States? For most of us, the answer is "never," and yet who is he compared to the God of this universe? The fact is, sometimes we forget who we're talking to.

Prayer is the art of communication, and I've yet to meet a girl who doesn't like to communicate. We talk to understand and to be understood. Talking to God is no different. We communicate to know him better and to tell him our requests. Prayer is key to establishing, strengthening, and nurturing our relationship with God.

Soulful Solutions

Ephesians 6:18—And pray in the Spirit on all occasions with all kinds of prayers and requests. With this in mind, be alert and always keep on praying for all the saints.

Now that you've got your belt, breastplate, shoes, shield, helmet, and sword, it may appear that you're ready for battle. But there's one important thing left to do; you must talk to the Commander in Chief. Military troops aren't ready to execute any exercise without explicit instructions from their leader. Communication plays a key role in carrying out a successful mission.

Our mission is life, and all the struggles that accompany it. Even when we're suited up in the armor of God and reading the Bible, it's crucial that we follow up with prayer. Communication is key to discerning truth, sharing the good news, enhancing our faith, and receiving insight into God's Word. Prayer gives life, sustains life, and enriches life. Prayer has perks.

Scripture It

Philippians 4:6 (CEV)—Don't worry about anything, but pray about everything. With thankful hearts offer up your prayers and requests to God.

Simply put, prayer is talking to God. Through prayer, we acknowledge his presence and strengthen our faith. In the most devastating of circumstances, when it seems all hope is lost, we still have prayer. And as we pray our faith will grow. Soon you'll be praying with a thankful heart, knowing that God not only hears but answers.

Prayer is an opportunity that should never be taken for granted. It needs to be carried out in a sincere fashion—we need to pray in style. Just as there are steps to follow for PERMS, there are also basic guidelines to prayer.

Way to PRAYS

In order to keep prayer in the proper perspective, so it's not just about everything I want, I follow this easy little acronym: **PRAYS**—Praise, Repent, Acknowledge, Yield, Silence. This simple reminder helps me pray effectively.

Step #1—Praise His Name

Hebrews 13:15—Through Jesus, therefore, let us continually offer to God a sacrifice of praise—the fruit of lips that confess his name.

"Dear God, I love you, I praise you, I worship you, I adore you, and I thank you for sending your Son to die that I might live. You're awesome!"

Begin your prayer by giving God a place of honor in your heart, soul, and mind. Praise not only elevates God, it also humbles us when we come before him. I often begin my prayer time with worship songs, singing directly to the One they were created for. Sometimes I even put a praise CD on and crank up the music to get myself started. The dictionary defines praise as: **to commend the worth of; to glorify God, as in song.** So start your prayer with style: **Raise your praise to the most high God!**

Step #2—Repent Your Sin

Proverbs 15:29—The LORD is far from the wicked, but he hears the prayer of the righteous.

"Lord, please forgive me for my sin. Help me to be aware of temptations, and when they come my way, please enable me to overcome them."

Each of us will sin every day of our lives but we must not let it separate us from God. God can't be a party to sin; he's perfect, holy, and sinless in every way. When sin creeps into our life, it pushes God out. So repent of your sin, asking God's forgiveness for anything you've done wrong. And make a conscious effort to pray throughout the day, asking forgiveness when you mess up.

Don't save up sin, allowing it to accumulate until it drives a wedge between you and God. That will only leave you wallowing in hopelessness. When you've really messed up, and you feel there is nowhere to turn—look up.

There's nothing you've done that God won't forgive if you just ask. And you can even solicit God's help when it comes to fighting sin. I ask him to make me acutely aware of temptation. When it creeps up on me, I instantly pray and ask for strength to beat the temptation.

To repent is defined as **to feel regret over (an error or sin), to change.** When we are truly remorseful, we can change and avoid making the same mistakes. As I see it there's only one way to really become a better person, and that is **to pray away sin every day!**

Step #3—Acknowledge His Faithfulness

Colossians 4:2—Devote yourselves to prayer, being watchful and thankful.

"Father, I thank you for answering specific requests, as well as helping me at home, work, and school. Thank you."

How would you feel if you had a friend that only came around when she needed something? And what if she didn't even bother to thank you after you helped her? I don't know about you, but I'd feel rather used. I wonder how God feels when we only talk to him when we want something, and then we don't even remember to thank him when we get it? Saying thank you is an important part of prayer. It allows you to acknowledge God's faithfulness, and it also increases your faith as you recognize answered prayers.

We have so much to be thankful for. Yet we often take it for granted, forgetting that we are nothing without God. A verse in Philippians says, "My God shall supply all your need," and God supplies way beyond true needs. We look at needs as CD players, televisions, telephones, computers, DVD players, video games, trendy clothing and shoes,

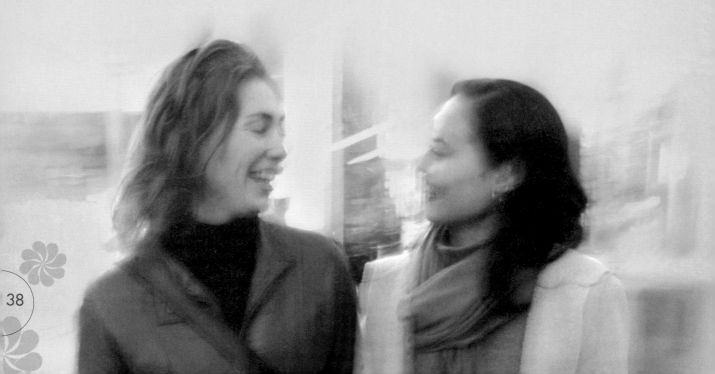

and cars. But in reality our only needs are God, water, food, shelter, and basic clothing. Do you see how much you have to be thankful for?

The definition of acknowledge is **to express thanks for.** According to Colossians we're supposed to do this with an attitude of thanksgiving, which is defined as **a formal public expression of thanks to God.** In other words, we're not only to thank God, but we are to openly acknowledge him. When was the last time you prayed and thanked God for your food while sitting in the school cafeteria? This simple act of thanksgiving shows God, yourself, and others that you acknowledge his goodness. **Dear God, for all you do I thank you!**

Step #4—Yield Your Requests

1 Peter 5:7—Cast all your anxiety on him because he cares for you.

> "Dear Lord, please hear my requests and answer them according to your plan. Thank you for hearing my heart and caring about me down to the very tiniest of details. I love you."

God cares about everything you care about. If you're worried about someone who's sick, God cares too. If you care about getting good grades in school, God does too. From your worries to your wants, God cares more than you could imagine. You're his daughter, and as your father, God wants to give you what's best for you. We just have to ask. His Word tells us in James 4:2, "You do not have, because you do not ask God."

When you make a request, it's important to yield it to God and not take it back. I have trouble with this. I'm guilty of casting my request to God and then reeling it right back in. I remember once when my brother took me fishing. He bought me a license, loaned me a rod and reel, and even stuck the worm on the hook. The only thing I had to do was cast it into the lake and wait. Waiting—that was the hard part. I grew impatient, bored, and frustrated waiting to reel in a fish. So I made up a game. I'd cast the line out and reel it back in, over and over, which made my brother crazy. He said, "You'll never catch anything if you keep pulling your line in. Cast it and leave it out there. Be patient, relax, and wait."

I hate waiting, even in my prayer life. So what do I do? I cast my prayer up and when I don't see an answer bobbing around in what I think is a timely manner, I take it back. Of course, after I work on my own solution for awhile, I discover it's hopeless and I cast it back to God. It's a game I shouldn't play. Instead, I should put my brother's advice to use: cast it, leave it, and patiently wait on God.

Yield means **to surrender,** and surrender means **to give up possession of.** We are to give up ownership of our prayer requests and never take them back. When you give something away it's no longer yours. So once you place your cares and concerns in God's hands, let go. **There's no order too tall, too great, too small. Our God and Father can handle them all!**

Step #5—Silence Yourself

Psalm 46:10—Be still, and know that I am God.

"Father, now I ask that you help me be silent and devote my attention entirely to you, so that I can hear your heart. In Jesus' name, Amen."

This is the toughest part of prayer for me—sitting silently and listening. And yet this is what we need. Have you ever gotten annoyed with someone who asked you a question and didn't have the decency to listen to your answer? It's rude. We don't like it when others disrespect us in that manner, and yet we have the audacity to treat God this way. How rude!

I'm horrible at sitting still; I fidget around like I've got ants in my pants. Silence and stillness are just not in my vocabulary, yet this is what God calls us to do. It's tough but it can be done. Set a timer or your alarm clock for five minutes, and then sit in silence, focused on God. Try not to let your mind wander, and if it does, simply refocus your attention on God. Sit and listen to what he wants to impress upon your heart. Silence yourself and listen to God.

Silence means **to be silent, still, noiseless.** Invest five minutes of silence with God, and I promise you'll reap the profits many times over. **Sit still to hear God's will.**

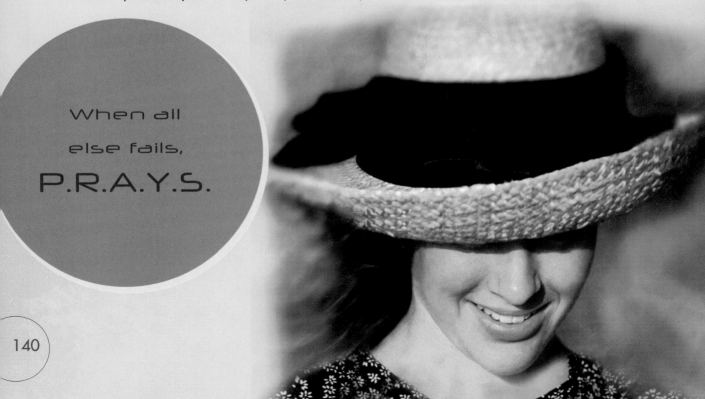

When all else fails, P.R.A.Y.S.

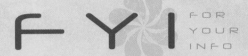

I've found that the best way to track prayer progress is in a prayer diary. It will help you focus on praise, be accountable for sin, recall reasons for thanks, and track prayer requests as well as their answers. It really is a fun, easy way to organize and get your prayer time under control.

Here's what you'll need:

1 three-ring binder (I like the kind with the see-through cover that you can decorate yourself)

5 dividers

Notebook paper and a pen or pencil

Label the first divider PRAISE—Use this section to record your praise to God.

Label the second divider REPENT—Use this section to admit your sin and repent.

Label the third divider ACKNOWLEDGE—Use this section to acknowledge God's goodness.

Label the fourth divider YIELD—Use this section to record your prayer requests.

Label the fifth divider SILENCE—Use this section to record what God says to you.

Set your notebook up with the dividers and notebook paper, and you're ready to start your prayer diary. Each day record the date and appropriate response in each section, skipping a line between entries in case you want to go back and add something later. In the YIELD section, you'll want to go back and record the date and answers to each specific request. Your prayer diary will help you develop stronger faith and establish a more exciting relationship with God.

Test It Out

In this chapter we've learned some very important advice about who we are (PERMS), and what we can become through prayer (PRAYS). We discovered that our self-esteem is wired by who we are physically, emotionally, relationally, mentally, and spiritually. And we've also seen how prayer can help you in each of those areas. Prayer transforms your outlook, making you feel better from the inside out. It helps you gain confidence in who you are through Christ. So put prayer into practice and become a Super Model who likes herself from the inside out.

Praise his name (Hebrews 13:15).

Repent your sin (Proverbs 15:29).

Acknowledge his faithfulness (Colossians 4:2).

Yield your requests to God (1 Peter 5:7).

Silence yourself, sit still, and listen to God (Psalm 46:10).

Super Models embrace themselves in prayer.

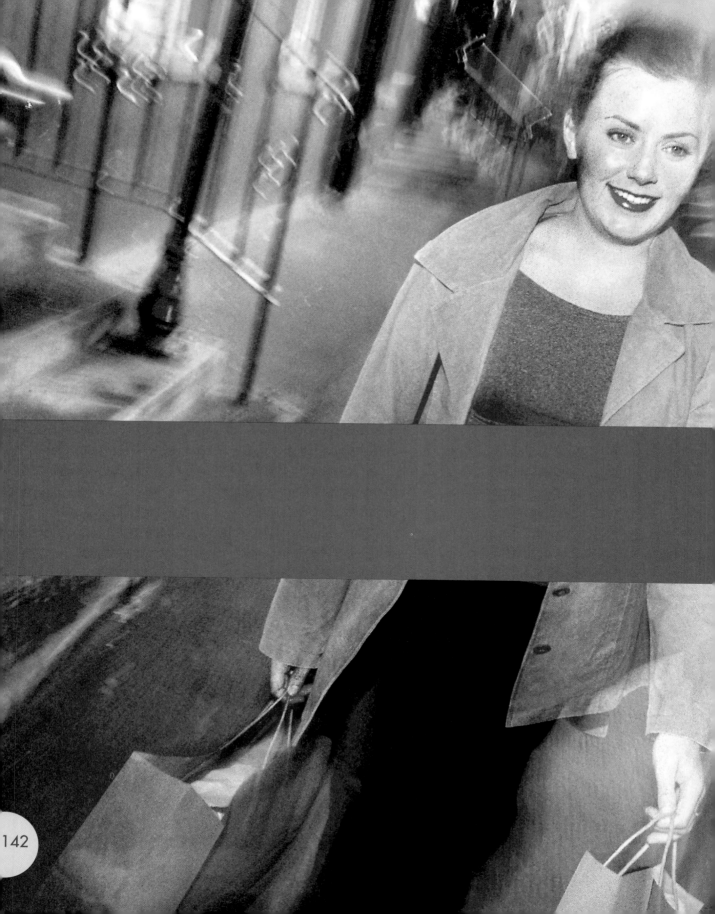

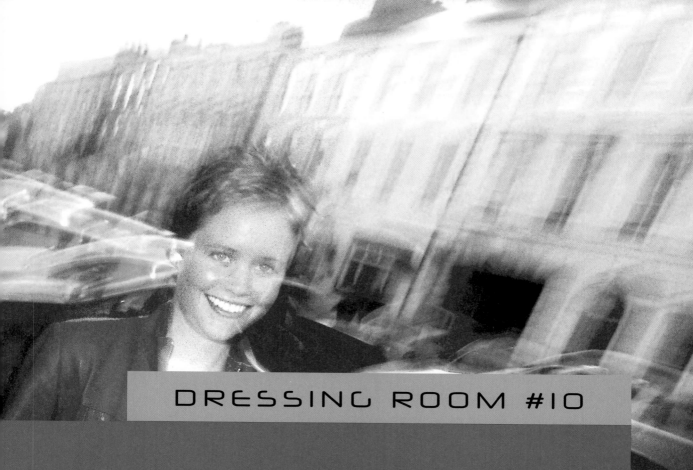

DRESSING ROOM #10

It's a Wrap

Part One—
Inquiring Minds Want to Know

So far, I've explained how to clean out the old, dress in the new, and tie it all together from the inside out through a relationship with Jesus Christ. I've given a lot of advice to you, so for this final chapter, I want to do something different. This chapter is totally dedicated to *you,* your thoughts, interests, and inquiring minds. After listening to advice from girls like you, I've decided to answer some of your most frequently asked questions. ❋ Questions help us learn, weigh the odds, and make sound decisions so that we can become the best that we can be. Not only that, but as a beauty bonus, I've run some of your questions past a panel of teenage girl experts—TEENAGE BOYS! So if you're ready, let's find answers for those questions!

All dressed up, places to go, things to do, and people to see—but there are so many things to learn in the process. There are questions that need answers, and responses that need questioning. So where do you find answers to the questions you didn't even know to ask?

Wise counsel is critical to growing up, but it's sometimes difficult to get the right answers from the right people at the right time. During the teenage years we often operate on a know-it-all attitude. But don't be an airhead. If you have questions, get answers. Part of dressing for success is beautifying your brain with brilliance.

Teenage girls from across the nation have asked the following questions via e-mail, survey, or face-to-face conversation. I've included my own answers and guy responses, which I gathered through polls and questionnaires.

Q. What should I wear on a date?

A. First, consider where you're headed. Are you going to a movie or are you going to the prom? The type of dress you choose—casual, formal, or somewhere in between—will be determined by the destination. Whatever you wear, dress with self-respect in mind. You'll be respected in the same manner in which you respect yourself.

Modesty
is the best
policy.

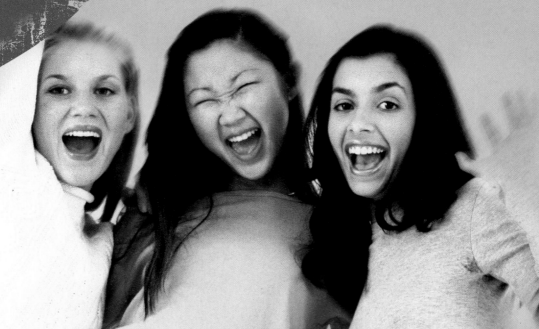

Guy Reply—

"Girls that dress loose on a date make me feel guilty because it makes me think about sex the whole time instead of focusing in on the girl so I can get to know her better. It also makes me feel sorry for her because she thinks that I won't like her unless she dresses that way." *Chris, VA*

Q. **How can you dress stylish when you're overweight?**

A. Being overweight can be quite a fashion predicament when you're trying to shop in the teenage department of most retail stores. For girls in general, one of the biggest fashion mistakes I see them make is wearing clothing that is too tight. Unfortunately, when you have extra pounds, they are amplified by wearing tight-fitting clothes. You actually look thinner in clothing that is slightly larger rather than clothing that is too small. I recommend that you wear a loose-fitting blouse that hangs straight down from your shoulders. This will help camouflage extra weight even if you wear it as a jacket over a form-fitting shirt. Also try wearing the same color from head to toe; this is more slimming than wearing different colors. For example, wear black pants and a black shirt to create a slimming vertical line, and then accessorize with a different color blouse as a jacket. Finally, try to lose the added weight; it will help you look and feel better emotionally and physically.

Q. **How should I dress for a job interview?**

A. You only get one opportunity to make a good first impression, and what better way to make a good impression than to dress well for an interview? The type of clothing you wear will be determined by the kind of job you apply for. Everyone should dress respectably and practice good personal hygiene, no matter what the job consists of. I asked a variety of managers (from fast food to retail) what they preferred *not* to see at an interview, and the common denominators were blue jeans and body piercing (other than the ears).

Q. **How can I dress nice and still be comfortable?**

A. Being comfortable is important, especially when you have to sit in school for seven hours a day. But dressing up a bit has been proven to increase your school performance. So is it possible to have it both ways? Absolutely. I recommend that you stay away from restrictive clothing, such as tight jeans, and avoid wearing anything that makes you feel dumpy, such as sloppy jeans or big slouchy T-shirts. Some great alternatives are stylish sweat suits, loose-fitting khakis, or a casual denim skirt.

Q. Do guys prefer dresses or pants?

A. I'll leave this one to the guys.

Guy Replies—

"I like when girls dress like girls instead of wearing guys clothes." *Ryan, NM*

"I don't care if they wear pants or dresses as long as they dress modestly." *Josh, NC*

"I like when girls dress attractive. I guess I notice girls more in dresses because you don't see them wear them too often." *Jeff, CA*

Q. How can I dress in style and be modest at the same time?

A. Keep yourself covered and don't cover yourself too tightly. Wear tank tops under low-cut shirts and don't wear tight pants; if you can see your panty line, they're too tight. If you wear dresses or skirts they should be a modest length (no shorter than three or four inches above your kneecap).

❋ Simple Solutions

Q. How can I get bloodstains (from my period) out of my clothes?

A. Attend to the stain as soon as possible. For outer garments such as pants or jeans, apply a laundry stain remover and vigorously scrub fabric back and forth between hands. Rinse with lukewarm water (don't use hot water because it sets stains). To remove stains from undergarments, soak in a mixture of $1/4$ cup hydrogen peroxide and 1 quart of water for thirty minutes and then rinse.

Q. How can I prevent buttons from falling off?

A. It seems like half the clothes we buy seem to lose their buttons. Here's a great solution that someone showed me. Dab a little nail glue or clear fingernail polish in the center of each button. This acts as an invisible thread sealer, keeping your buttons in place.

Q. How can I replace the pull-tab on the zipper of my favorite jeans?

A. Use a small safety pin or paper clip to replace the tab of any broken zipper pull.

Q. How long should I save receipts, and how can I easily keep track of them?

A. I save all my receipts in an envelope labeled "receipts" and I keep the envelope in my desk drawer. Depending on the item, I save receipts for up to a year or longer if I've purchased an extended warranty. If you're talking about clothing I keep the receipt at least until the first washing to make sure it doesn't fall apart in the process.

Q. I'm always losing earrings. How can I keep track of them?

A. A simple, inexpensive way to keep track of earrings is to separate them and store them in emptied egg cartons. Try using an empty film container to carry earrings (or loose change) in your purse, book bag, or gym bag.

Q. Is there any way to get wrinkles out of your clothes without ironing them?

A. Absolutely. You can either hang them in the bathroom while you're showering and steam them out, or you can throw them in the dryer with a damp towel (use spray bottle to spray the towel) and let them tumble for about 10–15 minutes.

Q. How can I pull clothes over my head without getting makeup on them?

A. Drape a silk scarf over your head and then slip the top on. This will keep your makeup on your face and off your clothes. Pack a scarf in your purse when you go shopping; the stores will love you for it.

Q. My white tops seem to turn yellow or gray after a while. Is there any way to turn them white again?

A. Wash whites in hot water using borax and your favorite laundry detergent.

Q. How can I make my dresser drawers smell good without buying expensive sachets?

A. You can spray an index card with your favorite perfume, use dryer sheets, or store a bar of fragrant soap in your dresser drawers. To scent your closet, step inside it to apply perfume; you'll smell good and the scent will linger long after you've left.

PICTURE IT 5

Q. Should I match my eye shadow to my eyes or to my clothes?

A. Never match your eye shadow to your eye color; your eyes will be lost in the monochromatic color scheme. Either compliment your eye color or the outfit you're wearing.

Q. How can I save money on a prom dress?

A. Try what my daughter and her girlfriends do: Have a dress swap. They borrow each other's dresses and then add new accessories such

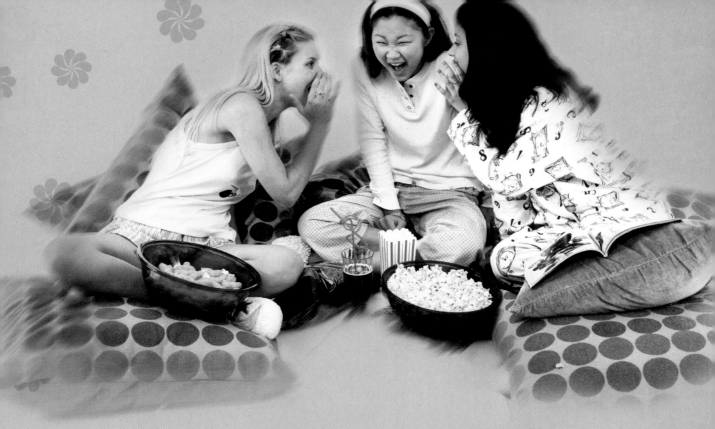

as jewelry, shoes, makeup, and hairdos. No one has ever noticed that they are wearing each other's dresses because each gal brings her own personal style to the outfit.

Q. How can I find a swimsuit that is right for my body type?

A. The most important factor to purchasing any swimsuit is modesty; leave something to the imagination. Next consider your body shape.

Pear Shape—The goal is to minimize your bottom and maximize your top.

Rectangle Shape—The goal is to visually create curves through the use of a printed fabric or the actual lines of the suit.

Apple Shape—The goal is to downplay your middle. Solid colors work best.

Hourglass Shape—The goal is to enhance your figure as well as support your breasts without exposing too much cleavage.

Wedge Shape—The goal is to create visual balance between your top and bottom.

Guy Reply—

"I'm more comfortable around a girl in a modest swimsuit because then I view her as a person and not an object of sex." *Matt, CA*

Q. How can I fix a snagged sweater?

A. Use a needle threader and pull the snag through to the inside of the sweater. Never cut the snag off because this will make a hole. If a sweater pills, use scissors and carefully cut them off.

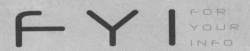

F Y I
FOR YOUR INFO

Here are answers to some of the questions that you specifically asked the guys.

Q. What do guys like the most in girls?

Guy Replies—

"A good personality and good sense of humor." Roger

"Honesty." Johnathon

"Someone easy to talk to with pretty eyes." Peter

Q. How do you treat a girl you're sincerely interested in?

Guy Replies—

"With respect." Paul

"The best way I can and with respect." Daniel

"Talk to her a lot." Joshua

Q. What is the one feature that makes a girl beautiful to you?

Guy Replies—

"Her eyes and her smile." Dave

"Her faith in God." Chris

"How she treats others." Ryan

Q. Do you prefer good looks or a great personality?

Guy Replies—

"Personality definitely." Eric

"Personality. If a girl is pretty but shallow I wouldn't be attracted to her. A good personality is the one thing that makes a girl beautiful to me." Allen

"Both." Scott

Q. Do you like the girl to pursue you or you to pursue the girl?

Guy Replies—

"I like to approach the girl first but I don't like it if she plays hard to get." James

"I like when the girl flirts with me first because I know she's interested." Mike

"I dunno. Depends on the girl." Adam

❋ What This Means 2U
Getting answers to your questions is extremely important. And there are many places you can find answers. Ask your parents, an older sibling, teachers, counselors, or youth workers. Surf the net, read a book, or write in to a magazine. *Brio* magazine (www.briomag.com) or *Beautiful Girl* magazine (www.beautifulgirlmagazine.com) are both great, safe places to start.

❧ Test It Out
When you ask questions, always check out your answers. There are a lot of people out there passing out bad information, and it's up to you to discern right from wrong. If something doesn't jive, then get a second opinion. One sure way to get the correct answers is to check them against the truth; God's absolute Truth. The truth is, when you're right with God, there's nothing wrong.

You Got Questions? I'll Get Answers
If you wish to be part of future polls and questionnaires, or if you have questions that need answers, write them down and email them to me at MakeOverMin@aol.com. Please indicate if this is a question for the boys or me. (Be aware that if it's for the guys it may be used as a survey question for future books.)

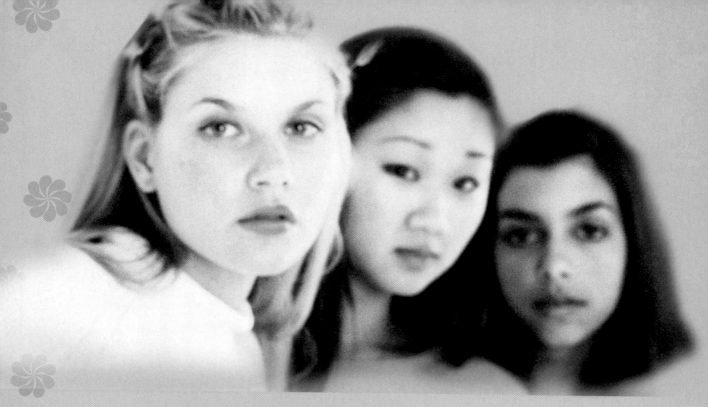

Part Two—Immortal Minds Want to Know

The answers to life's toughest questions can be solved by applying the **armor** of God.

We've learned about the armor of God and how it all fits, so now it's time to try it on for size. Our lives are filled with questions, but the biggest question is this: Will you live the kind of life that your armor can supply you with? ✳ Clothe yourself mind, body, and soul in God's armor so that you can stand against the devil's crafty tricks. You are no match for him alone, but when you utilize the armor and follow it up with prayer, Satan's as good as defeated. With God's armor on, we can answer any difficult question that he tries to confuse us with.

During my travels I've collected questions from teens, some of which no one else seems to know the answers to. I'm not some kind of know-it-all-genius, but I do know where to go for the true answers—God's Word.

As I prepared for this book I asked girls if there was anything in particular they wanted to know about the armor of God. Many girls asked how the armor of God applied to them directly, and others wanted to know which piece of armor is most important. Since we've already answered the first question throughout this book, let's use this chapter to answer the second question: "What is the most important piece of armor?"

Although each armor piece is necessary, it's the belt of truth that holds everything together. Truth is the single most important part of our protective gear. So now we're going to look for the truth. And where's the best place to find it? God's Word will give us the ironclad answers we need.

Soulful Solutions

Proverbs 20:18 (MESSAGE)—Form your purpose by asking for counsel, then carry it out using all the help you can get.

Q. Is anger wrong?

A. Anger is a natural emotion. We usually become angry when we've been wronged or know of someone else who has been mistreated. Even Jesus got angry when people used the temple as a store (Luke 19:45–46). The difference between good anger and bad anger is how you use it. For example, if drinking and driving makes you mad, join SADD (Students Against Drunk Driving). Use anger to prompt you toward good things, not bad things.

Armed with Answers—

Ephesians 4:26–27 (MESSAGE)—You do well to be angry—but don't use your anger as fuel for revenge. And don't stay angry. Don't go to bed angry. Don't give the Devil that kind of foothold in your life.

Prayer Pointers

Repent your wrong anger.

Ask for help controlling anger.

Q. How can I know God's plan and purpose for my life?

A. God will show you his plan through his Word, prayer, circumstances, and godly advice. He'll reveal what he has in store for you at precisely the right time. Seek wise counsel from your parents, grandparents, youth workers, and teachers. And remember, even when you're out on your own and all grown up, it's still cool to take advice.

Armed with Answers—

Proverbs 15:22 (MESSAGE)—Refuse good advice and watch your plans fail; take good counsel and watch them succeed.

Proverbs 3:5–6 (CEV)—With all your heart you must trust the LORD and not your own judgment. Always let him lead you, and he will clear the road for you to follow.

Prayer Pointers

Ask God to guide and direct you every day.

Ask him to show you his plans, and to help you do them.

Q. Is going to church really that important as long as I read the Bible and pray on my own?

A. Church is a great source of encouragement, where Christians can worship God, serve him, study Scripture, and pray for one another. Even though the church is made up of imperfect people like you and me, we can still learn from each other and hold each other accountable before God. So, the answer is, yes indeed, attending church is important.

Armed with Answers—

Hebrews 10:25 (CEV)—Some people have gotten out of the habit of meeting for worship, but we must not do that. We should keep on encouraging each other, especially since you know that the day of the Lord's coming is getting closer.

Prayer Pointers

Ask God to give you excitement about church.

Ask for godly friends who will worship with you.

Q. Will God keep forgiving me, even when I sin the same thing over and over again?

A. As long as we come to God and sincerely ask his forgiveness, the Bible says he will never refuse us or turn us away. If you have a problem with a particular sin, one that you just can't seem to shake, find someone to pray with and be accountable to.

Armed with Answers—

1 John 1:9 (CEV)—But if we confess our sins to God, he can always be trusted to forgive us and take our sins away.

Romans 8:38–39 (MESSAGE)—I'm absolutely convinced that nothing . . . absolutely *nothing* can get between us and God's love because of the way Jesus our Master has embraced us.

Prayer Pointers

Ask for forgiveness.

Ask for help to say "no" to temptation.

Q. My parents aren't Christians and they have asked me to do things that are wrong. What should I do?

A. The Bible tells us to obey our parents, but it also calls parents to teach their children godly ways. And God doesn't want any of us to sin. So how you respond will depend on what your parents are asking. For example, if they are asking you to lie by telling someone on the telephone that they are not home, you could simply say, "I'm sorry they aren't available right now" (which isn't a lie). But if they are asking you to do something that can't be done in an ethical way, such as stealing or selling drugs, respectfully tell them no. You don't want to destroy your relationship with your parents, because you may be the only one to share Christ with them. However, if you are in serious trouble, get help from someone else.

Armed with Answers—

Ephesians 6:1, 4 (MESSAGE)—Children, do what your parents tell you. This is only right. . . . Fathers, don't exasperate your children by coming down hard on them. Take them by the hand and lead them in the way of the Master.

Prayer Pointers

Ask for God's wisdom in the situation.

Pray for your parents to become Christians.

Scripture It

Proverbs 19:20 (CEV)—*Pay attention to advice and accept correction, so you can live sensibly.*

Q. **What does the Bible say about dating?**

A. The Bible does not address dating directly, but it does talk about relationships; your relationship with God, your parents, and even the opposite sex. In 2 Corinthians Paul tells us not to be unequally yoked with nonbelievers. This word picture brings to mind a pair of oxen, working together as a team and headed in the same direction. If you join a believer with a nonbeliever, one person is God-focused and the other isn't. There will be division and lack of understanding within the relationship as they head in different directions. So it's okay to have friends that don't know God, but don't attach yourself to them in a dating relationship or in marriage.

Armed with Answers—

2 Corinthians 6:14—Do not be yoked together with unbelievers. For what do righteousness and wickedness have in common? Or what fellowship can light have with darkness?

Prayer Pointers

Pray for your future husband.

Ask for patience to wait for the right man.

Q. **Since God made marijuana and the Bible doesn't say it's wrong, why shouldn't we smoke it?**

A. God doesn't address pot or other drugs in the Bible, but he does tell us to take care of our bodies, and to stay alert. God created plants

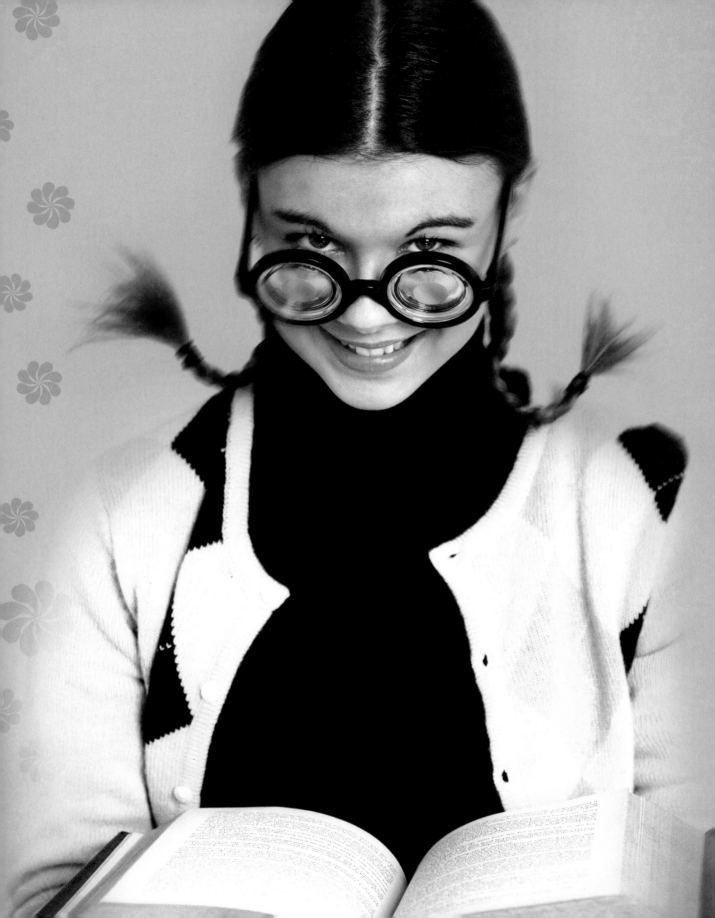

for many reasons, one of which is to be used as medicines. However, like so much in life, we've taken what God created for good and turned it into something evil. Many people use drugs as a way to escape reality. They become dependent on drugs instead of depending on God. The fact of the matter is, as a Christian your body is now a temple of the Holy Spirit. If you smoke marijuana, you're contaminating the temple.

Armed with Answers—

Titus 2:12 (NKJV)—Denying ungodliness and worldly lusts, we should live soberly, righteously, and godly in the present age.

1 Corinthians 6:19–20—Do you not know that your body is a temple of the Holy Spirit, who is in you, whom you have received from God? You are not your own; you were bought at a price. Therefore honor God with your body.

Prayer Pointers

Ask for courage to stand up against drug abuse.

Seek spiritual highs by growing in your relationship with God.

Q. Is homosexuality wrong?
A. Homosexuality, and all other forms of sexual immorality, are wrong; God calls it perversion (Lev. 18:6–23). God created sex for husband and wife, and homosexuality distorts that. Homosexuality is a sin, just as cheating, stealing, murder, and drug abuse are sins. And like drug abuse, it can be harmful and extremely addictive. The homosexual lifestyle *is* wrong, but so is condemning the homosexual. Don't fall prey to criticizing the sinner instead of the sin. We are to love and pray for the salvation of all people. If they accept Jesus, the Holy Spirit will convict them of their sin.

Armed with Answers—

Romans 1:26–27—God gave them over to shameful lusts. Even their women exchanged natural relations for unnatural ones. In the same way the men also abandoned natural relations with women and were inflamed with lust for one another. Men committed indecent acts with other men, and received in themselves the due penalty for their perversion.

1 Thessalonians 4:3–6 (CEV)—God wants you to be holy, so don't be immoral in matters of sex. Respect and honor your wife. Don't be a slave of your desires or live like people who don't know God. You must not cheat any of the Lord's followers in matters of sex.

Prayer Pointers

Ask for wisdom to confront homosexual sin.

Ask for help loving homosexuals.

Q. Is witchcraft real?

A. Witchcraft, fortune telling, wizardry, black magic—all are connected to Satan and the spiritual forces of this world (Eph. 6:12). People who practice witchcraft have joined forces with the devil and draw power from him. So stay away from anything that has to do with the occult; don't open yourself up to it in any way. Avoid Ouija boards. They're sold as a game, but they are really playing with the devil.

Armed with Answers—

Deuteronomy 18:11–12 (CEV)—And don't try to use any kind of magic or witchcraft to tell fortunes or to cast spells or to talk with spirits of the dead. The LORD is disgusted with anyone who does these things.

Prayer Pointers

Ask for protection from the attractions of witchcraft.

Pray for discernment in all you do.

Q. Is cybersex wrong even though you aren't really doing it?

A. Although the world says cybersex is no big deal, God says that any kind of sex outside of marriage is wrong. It doesn't matter if it's cybersex, oral sex, or casual sex. Sexual immorality of any kind can produce very damaging results both mentally and physically. Sex is both physical and mental, and the Bible says that if you even think about a guy in that way, you've already committed the sin in your heart. So that means that cybersex, or any kind of pornography, is wrong even if no physical touching takes place.

Armed with Answers—

1 Corinthians 6:13b, 18–20 (CEV)—We are not supposed to do indecent things with our bodies. We are to use them for the Lord who is in charge of our bodies. Don't be immoral in matters of sex. That is a sin against your own body in a way that no other sin is. You surely know that your body is a temple where the Holy Spirit lives. The Spirit is in you and is a gift from God. You are no longer your own. God paid a great price for you. So use your body to honor God.

Matthew 5:28 (CEV)—But I tell you that if you look at another woman [or man] and want her [or him], you are already unfaithful in your thoughts.

Prayer Pointers

Ask for protection from things you shouldn't see.

Seek to keep your thoughts pure.

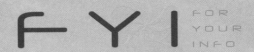

Guys have values too. When they are challenged to tell the truth, it's amazing how they really feel about some very personal issues.

Q. Would you date a non-Christian?

Guy Replies—

"No, because she might pull me down." Scott

"Maybe, but if I did it wouldn't be serious." Johnathon

"No, the Bible says not to." Will

Q. Will you marry a non-Christian?

Guy Replies—

"No, somewhere the Bible says not to be unequally yoked." Zach

"No, I want to marry someone who shares my same ideas." Paul

"No, because it never works when you think you'll change someone." Peter

Q. Would you prefer to marry a girl who has had sex with someone else or who saved herself just for you?

Guy Replies—

"I would rather have a girl that has only had sex with me because I would wonder if she was comparing me to other people." Nate

"I would like someone inexperienced, however if I really loved her I'd overlook her past." Matt

"I don't want to marry anyone that could have STDs." Adam

Q. When you see a girl dressed skimpy how does that make you feel?

Guy Replies—

"It makes me feel different, if you know what I mean." Josh

"Guilty for being so turned on." Tyler

"Like I shouldn't look, but I do anyway because it attracts my attention." Peter

Q. When you see a girl dressed skimpy, how does that make you feel towards the girl?

Guy Replies—

"She's easy and wants sex." Josh

"Slut comes to mind, but I also feel sorry for her." Tyler

"Not too highly of her, and that she's desperate for attention." Peter

Q. When you see a girl dressed skimpy, what do you think the girl is saying about herself?

Guy Replies—

"She does not feel good about herself." Josh

"Low self-esteem." Tyler

"Lack of self-respect. It's her only way of getting a guy's attention." Peter

Super Models **dress** themselves in the armor of God.

157

❋ What This Means 2U

God's armor isn't something you can purchase. But it was bought for a price—it cost Jesus his life. God gave his life so that you might live forever with him in heaven. The invitation is yours to accept, and once you R.S.V.P. you become part of a very posh party; you become a Christian.

As a Christian, you should strive to be more Christlike, and to attain this goal God has furnished you with a uniform—the armor of God. This armor provides a timeless wardrobe, and it'll help you face life's toughest questions with the truth.

❯Test It Out

We must dress our minds carefully. After all, that is where sin, doubt, and temptation are born, and our actions flow from our state of mind. So as you put your clothes on your body, I challenge you to prayerfully clothe your mind in the armor of God at the same time. And remember, the armor is not complete without prayer. Communication with God encourages us to dress for success in all we say and do.

Ask questions.

Research your answers when you're in doubt.

Make dressing in God's armor a routine habit.

Obligate yourself to becoming more Christlike.

Remember to always pray.

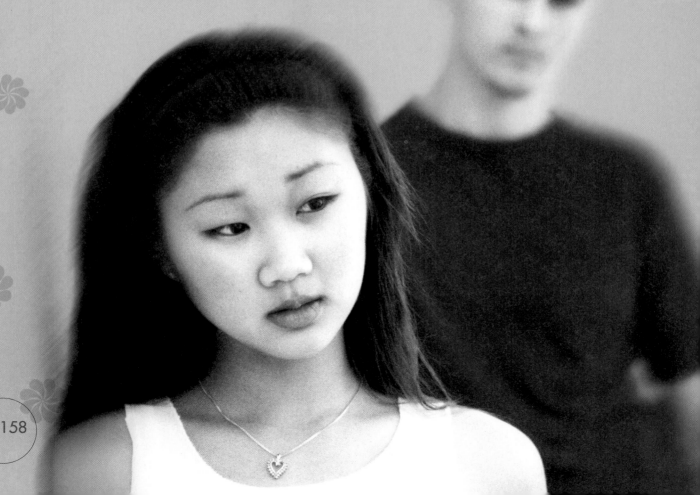

To Clothes

Wow! This is it. One final fashion farewell and we're finished.

Dressing from the inside out projects a great fashion image. What we wear on the outside is important to our modesty, self-esteem, and self-worth, but it all starts with a state of mind. Thinking positively of yourself will entice others to think of you that way too.

As a Christian, you are clothed in the Spirit of God. You are a princess, the daughter of the King of kings. People should see Jesus living in you, through the way you act, talk, and look. You never get a second chance to make a first impression, so make your first impression count for eternity. You might be the only living example of God that some people ever witness.

Getting dressed is not about designer labels, it's about the Designer of the universe—God—and how we apply him to our lives. The key to getting dressed, both body and soul, is linked to the clothesline of your heart through your relationship to Jesus Christ. Always dress with him in mind.

P.S. If you wish to be part of future polls or if you have any questions of your own, I can be reached at MakeOverMin@aol.com.

Tammy

Super Models adorn themselves in the full **armor** of God.

159

Many Thanks

I could not have written this book without many special people in my life encouraging me to be all that I can be from the inside out. I truly love and adore each one of you.

To my husband, Ed: You have set the standard of excellence among godly men of integrity. I love you, and I'm so blessed to have you love me and all my little quirks (like Christmas music in July).

To my favorite son, Matthew: You are truly a gift from God. I'm blessed to be your mom.

To my favorite daughter, Ashlee: You mirror what it is to be a Super Model from the inside out. I'm the luckiest mom in the whole wide world to have you as my girl.

To Dad and Mom: Your godly examples have changed lives for the better; especially those of your children.

To Florence Littauer: I couldn't have done any of this without your mentoring.

To Fred Littauer: Although you're no longer with us here on earth, your cheerful greetings will remain in our hearts.

To Art and Winnie Rorheim: Thanks for being obedient to God's calling. AWANA changed my life.

To my girlfriends who love me in spite of myself—Beth, Rose, Jo-Anne, Charlotte, and Ona: The book's finished, so let's go shopping. And lunch is on me!

To my lifelong friend, Diane: Thanks for the memories!

To all my friends at Baker Book House—Jennifer, Robin, Kristin, Twila, Karen S., Ruth, Dwight, Dave, Dan, Cheryl, Karen V., Rebecca, and Mike: Thank you for making my dream to touch the lives of teenage girls a reality.

To my panel of experts: Thanks for being good sports and answering the questionnaires to the truest of your ability.

To you my readers: Thank you for reading this book. I'd love to hear what you thought about it, and answer any questions you might have. E-mail me at MakeOverMin@aol.com.

And last but not least, God and Father, thank you for allowing me to be the pen in your hand. I dedicate this book to your plan and purpose.

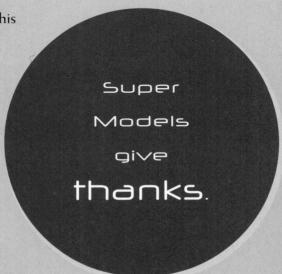

Super Models give **thanks.**

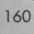